Lecture Notes in Computer Science   10883

Commenced Publication in 1973
Founding and Former Series Editors:
Gerhard Goos, Juris Hartmanis, and Jan van Leeuwen

More information about this series at http://www.springer.com/series/7412

Stefan Klein · Marius Staring
Stanley Durrleman · Stefan Sommer (Eds.)

Biomedical Image Registration

8th International Workshop, WBIR 2018
Leiden, The Netherlands, June 28–29, 2018
Proceedings

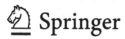 Springer

Editors
Stefan Klein ⓘ
Erasmus MC
Rotterdam
The Netherlands

Stanley Durrleman
Inria/ICM ARAMIS Lab
Paris
France

Marius Staring ⓘ
Leiden University Medical Center
Leiden
The Netherlands

Stefan Sommer ⓘ
University of Copenhagen
Copenhagen
Denmark

ISSN 0302-9743   ISSN 1611-3349   (electronic)
Lecture Notes in Computer Science
ISBN 978-3-319-92257-7   ISBN 978-3-319-92258-4   (eBook)
https://doi.org/10.1007/978-3-319-92258-4

Library of Congress Control Number: 2018944383

LNCS Sublibrary: SL6 – Image Processing, Computer Vision, Pattern Recognition, and Graphics

Printed on acid-free paper

This Springer imprint is published by the registered company Springer International Publishing AG
part of Springer Nature
The registered company address is: Gewerbestrasse 11, 6330 Cham, Switzerland

Preface

The 8th International Workshop on Biomedical Image Registration (WBIR 2018, https://wbir2018.nl) was held in Leiden, The Netherlands, June 28–29, 2018. The workshop brought together leading researchers in the area of biomedical image registration to present and discuss recent developments and methodology in the field. WBIR 2018 was jointly organized by the image registration groups from Erasmus MC, Rotterdam, and LUMC, Leiden. The workshop included both oral and poster presentations in a single track, two keynote lectures, an image registration challenge, a post-conference hackathon, and ample opportunities for discussion.

Preceding editions of WBIR have been running mostly standalone as a 2-day workshop, alternating between U.S. and European locations: Bled, Slovenia (1999); Philadelphia, USA (2003); Utrecht, The Netherlands (2006); Lübeck, Germany (2010); Nashville, USA (2012); London, UK (2014); and Las Vegas, USA (2016).

The WBIR 2018 proceedings, published in the *Lecture Notes in Computer Science*, were established through a rigorous peer-review process in a double-blind fashion by at least three members of the Program Committee. The international Program Committee consisted of 31 senior scientists in the field of medical image registration. From a total of 17 submissions, 11 were selected for oral or poster presentation. This year, three papers were on the topic of sliding motion, three on groupwise image registration, one on acceleration, and four on applications and evaluation. New to WBIR, this year we invited 1-page abstract submissions in addition to full-paper submissions. This gave scientists the opportunity to present early work and to get feedback from conference attendees on recently published or submitted journal papers not presented previously. A total of 16 abstracts were submitted, which do not appear in the proceedings, but were presented at the conference.

Three excellent keynote speakers enriched the program. Prof. Dr. Jan-Jakob Sonke spoke about the utilization of image registration in the context of adaptive radiation therapy. Prof. Dr. Max Welling spoke about graph neural networks and related attention mechanisms for use in medical imaging. Prof. Dr. Julia Schnabel postulated that our field is currently finding itself at the cross-roads under the thought-provoking title "Is image registration a solved problem?". The program incorporated presentation of the design and results of the Continuous Registration Challenge, a new idea for benchmarking medical image registration algorithms. A post-conference hackathon, organized in collaboration with the Insight Toolkit (ITK) community and Kitware (Matt McCormick), greatly stimulated the implementation of ideas emerging from the workshop and enabled integration of new registration methods in the challenge.

Many contributed to the success of WBIR 2018. In particular, we would like to thank the members of the Program Committee for their work that assures the high quality of the workshop. Dr. Oleh Dzyubachyk is acknowledged as the proceedings editor, and Sahar Yousefi, MSc, as the webmaster. We also thank Inria, Quantib and the Netherlands Organisation for Scientific Research (NWO) for their financial support, and the MICCAI Society for their endorsement. Finally, we would like to thank all participants of WBIR 2018 for their contributions and discussions. We hope you had a great time in Leiden!

June 2018

Stefan Klein
Marius Staring
Stanley Durrleman
Stefan Sommer

Organization

WBIR 2018 was jointly organized by the image registration groups from Erasmus MC, Rotterdam, and LUMC, Leiden.

General Chairs

Stefan Klein   Erasmus MC, The Netherlands
Marius Staring   Leiden University Medical Center, The Netherlands

Program Chairs

Stanley Durrleman   Inria/ICM ARAMIS Lab, France
Stefan Sommer   University of Copenhagen, Denmark

Local Organization

Oleh Dzyubachyk   Leiden University Medical Center, The Netherlands
Sahar Yousefi   Leiden University Medical Center, The Netherlands

Program Committee

Gary Christensen	Iowa Institute for Biomedical Imaging, USA
Olivier Commowick	Inria, France
Adrian Dalca	Massachusetts Institute of Technology, USA
Benoit Dawant	Vanderbilt University, USA
Ali Gholipour	Harvard Medical School, USA
Ender Konukoglu	ETH-Zurich, Switzerland
Sebastian Kurtek	Florida State University, USA
Christian Ledig	Imperial College London, UK
Marco Lorenzi	Inria, France
Andreas Maier	Friedrich-Alexander Universität, Germany
Stephen Marsland	Massey University, New Zealand
Matt McCormick	Kitware Inc., USA
Marc Modat	University College London, UK
Kensaku Mori	Nagoya University, Japan
Wiro Niessen	Erasmus Medical Center, The Netherlands
Marc Niethammer	University of North Carolina at Chapel Hill, USA
Bartłomiej Papież	University of Oxford, UK
Josien Pluim	Technical University Eindhoven, The Netherlands
Kilian Pohl	SRI International, USA
Karl Rohr	University of Heidelberg, Germany

Daniel Rueckert   Imperial College London, UK
Benoit Scherrer   Harvard Medical School, USA
Julia Schnabel   King's College London, UK
Dinggang Shen   University of North Carolina, USA
Aristeidis Sotiras   University of Pennsylvania, USA
Colin Studholme   University of Washington, USA
Lisa Tang   The University of British Columbia, Canada
Matthew Toews   Ecole de Technologie Superieure, Canada
Carole Twining   University of Manchester, UK
Jef Vandemeulebroucke   Vrije Universiteit Brussel, Belgium
Tom Vercauteren   University College London, UK

Contents

Applications and Evaluation

Sliding Motion

An Inhomogeneous Multi-resolution Regularization Concept for Discontinuity Preserving Image Registration

Christoph Jud[(✉)], Robin Sandkühler, and Philippe C. Cattin

Department of Biomedical Engineering, University of Basel, Allschwil, Switzerland
christoph.jud@unibas.ch

Abstract. Sliding organs pose challenges in the registration of dynamic medical images because the smoothness criterion which is commonly assumed over the whole image domain does not apply at the sliding interfaces. In this case, image registration methods have to cope with local discontinuities in the correspondence map. We present a new registration methodology based on a multi-resolution transformation model which is defined as a directed acyclic graph. The graph's edges connect consecutive resolution levels enabling to inhomogeneously pass displacements through to higher levels. Thus, they are well suited to cope with local discontinuities while aiming at smooth correspondence maps. We introduce three regularization terms which operate on the graph. A total variation term ensuring discontinuity preserving smoothness, a sparsity term on zero edge-weights to prevent trivial solutions and a term which prefers transformations which are explained in lower resolution levels. For an early proof of concept we analyze the registration performance of our method on synthetic 2D data and on a 2D slice of the POPI model.

1 Introduction

Temporally resolved medical images have gained a lot of attention in the past years. They show promise because the motion information contained therein allows to draw conclusions about the anatomical dynamics. An integral part for extracting the motion from such images forms the process of finding corresponding structures of successive images which is referred to as image registration. As image registration is a nonlinear ill-posed problem regularization is inevitable to attain plausible correspondence. Smoothness of the correspondence map as an additional assumption is the most common regularization. It can be obtained by mainly three mutually non-exclusive ways. (I) Smoothness is implicitly derived by *multi-resolution optimization* [6,17]. (II) In addition to image similarities a smoothness measure on the correspondence map is optimized e.g. the *diffusion regularization* [8,18] and/or (III) the correspondence map is defined in a smooth basis e.g. a *b-spline basis* [3,13].

In this paper, we present a new non-parametric formulation for image registration which is targeted to the case where organs slide along each other, whose

S. Klein et al. (Eds.): WBIR 2018, LNCS 10883, pp. 3–12, 2018.
https://doi.org/10.1007/978-3-319-92258-4_1

sliding interfaces locally contradict global smoothness assumptions. The novelty of our approach lies in the explicit treatment of local discontinuities which are built into the main objective. Specifically, in our method, we achieve smooth correspondence maps with point (I) and (II). We build (I) a hierarchy of displacement fields with resolution levels starting from one pixel (rigid translation) up to a displacement field that has the resolution of the images. Going up the hierarchy, the degrees of freedom is increased from level to level which gradually relaxes the influence of a level on the smoothness in the last level. To tackle discontinuities, we integrate a weighted propagation of displacements through the hierarchy in form of a directed acyclic graph (see Fig. 1). The weights are in the interval of $[-1, 1]$, thus, a displacement can be directly passed through (homogeneous case: weight = 1), it can be consumed (static and dynamic structure: weight = 0) or its direction can be inverted (dynamic structures moving in opposing directions: weight = -1). In addition, we introduce (II) a total variation smoothness term considering the total variation on each level. It is formulated such that it notably accounts for the weighted propagation in order to prevent total variation penalties across sliding interfaces. Furthermore, we do an L1 regularization on the weights and an L2 regularization on the displacements.

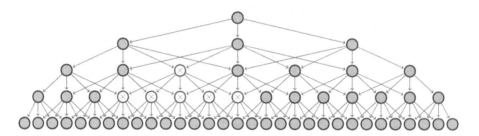

Fig. 1. Transformation model visualized as a directed acyclic graph. The nodes define the displacement at a certain position and the edges are the weights for the weighted propagation of the displacement down the displacement field hierarchy. The bottom level has the pixel size of the images. In blue and highlighted with crosses a neighborhood of a node is outlined. Each node has a bias which can initiate a displacement. (Color figure online)

Nonparametric image registration has been widely studied for more than two decades. Starting in the 90' [1,18] a lot of advanced approaches have been successfully applied to medical images. For a comprehensive review about image registration methods we refer to [16,21]. For methods which particularly address the sliding organ problem there are major categories of approaches. In [12,15], the registration task is divided into image regions segmenting the sliding parts in the image. The resulting correspondence map yields a composition of the registered regions. However, the sliding interfaces have to be known in advance. Various approaches [2,3,9,10,14] rely on local image features as e.g. image gradients, to identify the sliding interfaces and to relax the regularization across the interfaces. The implicit assumption made in these approaches is, that the sliding interfaces are located at high image gradients. For abdominal images, this is true for the lung and its sliding interface to the thoracic cavity. Nonetheless, it does not hold for sliding interfaces in general as e.g. the interface between the liver and the thoracic cavity. In [5,11], the sliding interfaces are derived by motion segmentation of the spatial transformation. The interfaces found are gradually refined during optimization based on the current correspondence map. To reach a stable convergence, however, remains challenging as the registration parameters and the motion segmentation are treated independently in the optimization. To avoid alternated optimization, in [4], motion segmentation is performed implicitly in the regularization term. No regional constraint on the segmentation was integrated though. In [3,22], sparsity is regularized to become robust against abrupt changes in the correspondence. However, the sliding interfaces are not explicitly considered.

Expressing discontinuities for the sliding interfaces requires high degrees of freedom which has to be trade-off against smoothness. It has been shown that starting with low degrees of freedom and successively adding more and more during optimization is advantageous to reach good optima [7]. This is why hierarchical image registration has found its way into most of the registration methods. However, only few approaches simultaneously optimize the full hierarchy of resolution levels at once [17,19] and they do not address sliding interfaces. In addition, it is not clear how to pass discontinuities contained in one level upwards the resolution hierarchy without an appropriate propagation.

The contribution of this paper is as follows. We present a concept of a transformation model which is flexible enough to express discontinuities and simultaneously can handle smooth regions on multiple scales. We implement it with a graph-based multi-resolution displacement field with a closely connected total variation regularizer which operates on the graph. Furthermore, we add an L1 penalty on the graph weights and an L2 penalty on the displacements. We show first results on synthetic 2D images and on a 2D slice of the POPI model [20] as an early proof of concept.

2   Method

A single-level displacement field as a transformation model where each pixel in the image domain can be transformed independently would not have any constraints, thus, discontinuous transformations could be well described. The same holds for a hierarchy of displacement fields. So, what is the motivation behind a hierarchy of displacement fields? Multi-grid methods found the way from general mathematical programming [7] to image registration methods [17]. Optimizing coarse approximation of a problem first and gradually refining the approximation during optimization has the effect of (I) smoothing the objective function and (II) reducing the sensitivity of the initialization to local minima. For common image registration objectives that means that the image gradient for a parameter in a coarser level is integrated over a larger domain than for one on the level of the image resolution which results in the effect of (I) and (II). For the sliding organ problem, however, gradients of opposing sides of sliding interfaces may cancel out each other. Therefore, we propose the weighted propagation to higher levels where the domain which is influenced by a parameter can be constrained.

2.1   Transformation Model

Let $\mathcal{X} := \{x_i\}_{i=1}^n$ be a set of n points lying on a regular grid and covering the joint image domain of the reference and target image $I_R, I_T : \mathcal{X} \to \mathbb{R}$ which map the d-dimensional input $\mathcal{X} \subset \mathbb{R}^d$ to intensity values. Let further $f : \mathcal{X} \to \mathbb{R}^d$ transform the reference coordinate system.

Image registration can be formulated as an optimization problem:

$$f_* := \arg\min_f \frac{1}{|\mathcal{X}|} \sum_{x \in \mathcal{X}} \mathcal{L}(I_R(x + f(x)), I_T(x)) + \eta \mathcal{R}[f, \mathcal{X}], \qquad (1)$$

where f_* is a minimizer of Eq. 1, $\mathcal{L}$ is a loss-function, $\mathcal{R}$ a regularization term weighted with the hyper-parameter η and $|\cdot|$ the cardinality of a set. Throughout the paper, we use the squared difference loss $\mathcal{L}(x, x') := (x - x')^2$. The regularization term $\mathcal{R}$ is explained in Sect. 2.2. The transformation f is defined to have a graph structure with several levels. Each level of the graph represents a different resolution, where the first level defines a coarse and the last a fine one. During minimization, the finer levels are successively added for the optimization and simultaneously optimized with the coarser levels.

Definition of the Graph. Let the transformation f be a directed acyclic graph having L levels, where each level l has N_l nodes $\{c_i^l\}_{i=1}^{N_l}$. Let the nodes be connected with directed edges $\phi(w_{ji}^{l-1}) \in [-1, 1], w_{ji}^{l-1} \in \mathbb{R}$ connecting the j-th node of level $l - 1$ with the i-th node of level l, where ϕ is a *logistic* function. We define the value of a node as

$$c_i^l = s^l b_i^l + \frac{1}{|\mathcal{B}_i^l|} \sum_{j \in \mathcal{B}_i^l} \phi(w_{ji}^{l-1}) c_j^{l-1}, \qquad (2)$$

where the root node $c_1^0 = s^0 b_1^0$, the biases $b_i^l \in \mathbb{R}^d$ and the scales $s^l \in \mathbb{R}_+$. The index set $\mathcal{B}_i^l$ contains the indices of the neighboring nodes $c_j^{l-1} \in \mathbb{R}^d$ (in the preceding level) of a node c_i^l. Nodes in the highest level $f(x_i) := c_i^{L-1}$ define the spatial transformation of f.

The number of nodes per level $N_l = \left(2 \sqrt[d]{N_{l-1}} + 1\right)^d$ and $N_0 = 1$ (see Fig. 1 for a 1D example). Each node c_i^l within the joint image region has a position in the image which corresponds to an $x_j^{L-1} \in \mathcal{X}$ where the spacing between nodes is the spacing of the preceding level divided by two. The root node c_1^0 is placed in the center of $\mathcal{X}$. We only consider edges w_{ji}^{l-1} which connect nodes c_j^{l-1} with *neighboring* nodes c_i^l denoted as $j \in \mathcal{B}_i^l$. We define the neighborhood of a node by considering ± 2 nodes in each space dimension resulting in a maximum size of the neighborhood of 5^d nodes. For regularization purposes (see Sect. 2.2) we set the scale values $s^l = 2^l$.

Logistic Function. To complete the definition of the transformation f we choose the following somewhat non-standard "logistic" function

$$\phi(w) := \sin(w) \tag{3}$$

because of several advantages. It maps each value into the desired interval $[-1, 1]$ and has gradients between $[-1, 1]$. A vanishing gradient of 0 is only attained at points $\pi/2 + k\pi$, for $k \in \mathbb{Z}$. Compared to the sigmoid function, where large steps lead to saturation, hitting vanishing gradients by chance is unlikely using the sine function.

2.2   Regularization

In the following, we construct three different regularization terms for the hierarchical transformation model. The TV-regularizer $\mathcal{R}_s$ which favors piece-wise smooth transformations, the sparsity regularizer $\mathcal{R}_w$ which penalizes weights which deviate from the values -1 and 1 and the bias regularizer $\mathcal{R}_b$ which favors transformations explained in lower levels by penalizing the magnitude of the biases. Finally, we replace the regularization term of Eq. 1 by

$$\mathcal{R}[f] := \eta_s \mathcal{R}_s[f] + \eta_w \mathcal{R}_w[f] + \eta_b \mathcal{R}_b[f] \tag{4}$$

with the hyper-parameters η_s, η_w and η_b.

TV Regularization with Edge Consideration. To regularize for smooth transformations, neighboring displacements which are similar should be desirable. This can be expressed by $\|c_i^l - c_j^l\|$ for neighboring c_i^l and c_j^l. We modify the norm to account for nodes which are located on opposing sides of sliding interfaces by defining the TV regularizer as:

$$\mathcal{R}_s = \sum_{l=1}^{L-1} \sum_{i=1}^{N_l} \sum_{j \in \mathcal{B}_i^l} \sum_{k \in (\mathcal{B}_i^l \cap \mathcal{B}_j^l)} \underbrace{\left\| \phi(w_{ki}^{l-1}) c_i^l - \phi(w_{kj}^{l-1}) c_j^l \right\|_\epsilon}_{\mathcal{C}} \underbrace{\left\| \phi(w_{ki}^{l-1}) \phi(w_{kj}^{l-1}) \right\|_\epsilon}_{\mathcal{W}},$$

where $\|x\|_\epsilon := \sqrt{x^T x + \epsilon}$. The special form of $\mathcal{C}$ with the factors ϕ is motivated as follows. If c_i^l and c_j^l are located on opposing sides of a sliding interface the contribution of the norm to the regularization term should be neglected. This can be achieved in two ways: if one node belongs to a static and the other to a dynamic structure the weights can be set to zero ($\mathcal{W} = 0$). If the nodes belong to distinct dynamic structures which slide along each other in opposite direction, the influence of the norm can be reduced by setting the weights for one node to 1 and for the other to -1. To summarize, the impact of the node c_i^l to $\mathcal{R}_s$ can be reduced by either aligning its neighboring nodes c_j^l (possibly in opposite direction) or by setting the weights connecting the two nodes over nodes in the preceding level to $\phi(w_{ki}^{l-1}) = \phi(w_{kj}^{l-1}) = 0$. Note that the first sum starts with level 1 as level 0 does not have any neighboring nodes on the same level. We simplify notation and omit the normalization factors of the inner three sums.

Sparsity Regularization on Edges. The piece-wise smoothness of R_s is enforced by the TV norm of neighboring nodes, however, the impact of this norm can be canceled out by the weights. One solution to minimize R_s is to set all weight parameters to $\pm\frac{\pi}{2}$ such that the weights $\phi(w) = 0$. We prevent such trivial solutions by an additional term R_w which penalizes weights deviating from the value ± 1.

$$R_w = \sum_{l=1}^{L-1}\sum_{i=1}^{N_l}\sum_{j\in\mathcal{B}_i^l} \frac{2}{\pi}\min\left(\left|\frac{\pi}{2} - w_{ji}^{l-1}\right|, \left|-\frac{\pi}{2} - w_{ji}^{l-1}\right|\right), \tag{5}$$

where R_w is further normalized by the number of considered weights. In Fig. 2, the influence of a weight parameter to the regularizer R_w is plotted.

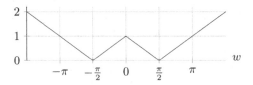

Fig. 2. Contribution of a weight to the regularization term R_w.

Regularization of Biases. As displacements are propagated upwards through the hierarchy of displacement fields, lower levels have a stronger influence on the smoothness of the final transformation i.e. the highest resolution level. Hence, favoring biases in lower levels directly means that smooth transformations are preferred. Therefore, we add a third regularization term

$$R_b = \sum_{l=0}^{L-1}\sum_{i=1}^{N_l}\|b_i^l\|^2, \tag{6}$$

where R_b is further normalized by the number of considered biases. Because the biases b_i^l are scaled with s^l, whose values decrease going up the hierarchy, the value of R_b can be reduced by explaining transformations with biases in lower levels.

3   Results

We evaluate our new hierarchical registration method (HReg) on two synthetic datasets to investigate hypothetical sliding organ boundaries. We compare our method to the sparse kernel machine (SKM) [3] based on the ground truth correspondence which is known in these examples. Furthermore, we show a qualitative result on a 2D slice of the 4DCT POPI model to verify a meaningful registration performance on biomedical data. In all experiments, we calculate analytical derivatives with respect to the biases and the weight parameters and minimize with an LBFGS optimizer including line search. For the sparsity regularizer $\mathcal{R}_w$, we use the sub-gradient of zero at values $w = \pm\frac{\pi}{2}$ and $w = 0$. The biases and weight parameters are initialized to zero and $\frac{\pi}{6}$ respectively.

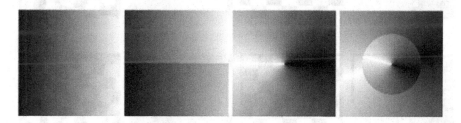

Fig. 3. Synthetic reference and target images. left: shift example, right: circle example.

Synthetic Examples. In the *shift* example, the shadings in the upper and lower part are shifted by 12 pixels in opposite directions between the target and reference image (c.f. Fig. 3). In the *circle* example, $I_R(x) = \frac{x \times e_1}{\pi}$, where e_1 is a unit vector. The inner and outer part are rotated by 15° in opposite directions between the target and reference image. The images in both examples have a size of 120 × 120 px and 7 graph-levels where used (127 × 127 px). As an evaluation measure, we define the error to the ground truth displacement field f_{gt} as $E[f, f_{gt}] := |\mathcal{X}|^{-1} \sum_{x \in \mathcal{X}} \|f(x) - f_{gt}(x)\|$.

Table 1. Ground truth difference $E[f, f_{gt}]$ [px] (*init* stands for the initial difference.)

	init	SKM	HReg
Shift	12	5.35	5.23
Circle	12	1.95	1.60

We manually tuned the hyper-parameters to starting values $\eta_s = \eta_w = \eta_b = \mathcal{D}[f_{\text{init}}] \cdot 10^{-2}$ for the *shift* and $\eta_s = \eta_w = \eta_b = \mathcal{D}[f_{\text{init}}] \cdot 10^{-3}$ for the *circle* experiment where $\mathcal{D}[f_{\text{init}}]$ is the integrated loss-function for the initial transformation f_{init}. The L1 regularization weight of the SKM was set for the three scale levels to $\{10^{-6}, 10^{-7}, 10^{-8}\}$. The sliding interfaces along the shift and circle respectively are well registered by HReg (see Fig. 4). There are remaining registration artifacts in the rotation center and the left and right side of the sliding interface. The resulting error $E[f, f_{gt}]$ of our method compared to the SKM method is similar (c.f. Table 1). Although, the SKM method achieved similar registration performance the correspondence map is smooth across the sliding interfaces.

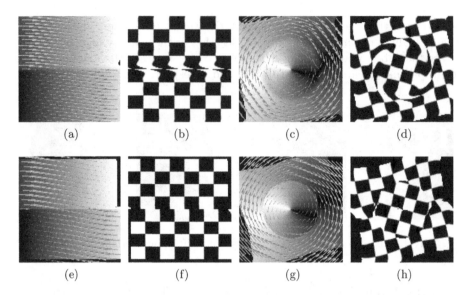

Fig. 4. Results of synthetic experiments (top row SKM, bottom row HReg). (a, c, e, g) warped reference where the final f_* is visualized with arrows, (b, d, f, h) checkerboard warped by the final f_*.

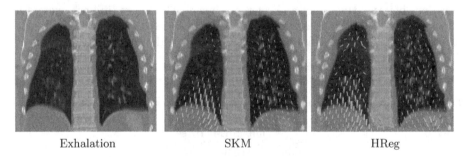

Exhalation   SKM   HReg

Fig. 5. Experiment with a slice of the POPI model. The displacement field is visualized as arrows colored in yellow. The background image is the warped inhalation slice. (Color figure online)

POPI Slice. For a qualitative evaluation, we register an inhalation and the corresponding exhalation slice of the 4DCT POPI model [20]. We re-sampled the images to a size of 125×103 px and used 7 levels in the transformation f. We manually set the hyper-parameters to $\eta_s = \mathcal{D}[f_{\text{init}}]$, $\eta_w = \mathcal{D}[f_{\text{init}}] \cdot 10^{-1}$, $\eta_b = \mathcal{D}[f_{\text{init}}] \cdot 10^{-4}$. When adding levels in the optimization the parameter η_s is changed to satisfy $\eta_s^{(l)} \mathcal{R}_s[f_*^{(l)}] = \eta_s^{(l+1)} \mathcal{R}_s[f_{\text{init}}^{(l+1)}]$ where the superscripts indicate how many levels are optimized. Thus, $f_*^{(l)}$ indicates the resulting minimizer f_* after optimizing with l levels and $f_{\text{init}}^{(l+1)}$ the initial transformation when starting the optimization with $l + 1$ levels. For the SKM method, we generated a *weight* image $I_w = -I_T$ which is further scaled to the interval $[0.1, 1]$. SKM and HReg perform on par looking at the registration result in Fig. 5. The weight image provided to the SKM, however, has the effect that the lower vertebrae are better mapped than in HReg. HReg in turn, better registers the inner part of the left lung.

4 Conclusion

We have proposed a new registration methodology targeted to the sliding organ problem. It is based on a hierarchical transformation model which has the form of a directed acyclic graph. The introduced regularization, which operates on this graph, is able to tackle the contradicting requirements on the correspondence map to be mostly smooth and to contain local discontinuities at sliding boundaries. We have analyzed the performance of our method on synthetic 2D registration examples and could show that compared to the SKM method, sliding interfaces are well registered. Finally, we have provided promising results on a 2D slice of the POPI model. Nevertheless, further investigations and tests are required for the individual components of the method which is planned for the future. As we have shown a proof of concept, we believe our method provides a rich framework for image registration problems with inhomogeneous smoothness requirements.

References

1. Bajcsy, R., Kovačič, S.: Multiresolution elastic matching. Comput. Vis. Graph. Image Process. **46**(1), 1–21 (1989)
2. Heinrich, M.P., Jenkinson, M., Brady, M., Schnabel, J.A.: MRF-based deformable registration and ventilation estimation of lung CT. IEEE Trans. Med. Imaging **32**(7), 1239–1248 (2013)
3. Jud, C., Möri, N., Cattin, P.C.: Sparse kernel machines for discontinuous registration and nonstationary regularization. In: Proceedings of the IEEE Conference on Computer Vision and Pattern Recognition Workshops, pp. 9–16 (2016)
4. Jud, C., Sandkühler, R., Möri, N., Cattin, P.C.: Directional Averages for motion segmentation in discontinuity preserving image registration. In: Descoteaux, M., Maier-Hein, L., Franz, A., Jannin, P., Collins, D.L., Duchesne, S. (eds.) MICCAI 2017. LNCS, vol. 10433, pp. 249–256. Springer, Cham (2017). https://doi.org/10.1007/978-3-319-66182-7_29
5. Kiriyanthan, S., Fundana, K., Majeed, T., Cattin, P.C.: Discontinuity preserving image registration through motion segmentation: a primal-dual approach. Comput. Math. Methods Med. **2016**, 20 (2016). Article ID 9504949
6. Lester, H., Arridge, S.R.: A survey of hierarchical non-linear medical image registration. Pattern Recogn. **32**(1), 129–149 (1999)
7. Mendonca, M.W.: Multilevel Optimization: convergence theory, algorithms and application to derivative-free optimization. Ph.D. thesis, Phd thesis, Facultés Universitaires Notre-Dame de la Paix, Namur, Belgium (2009)
8. Modersitzki, J.: Numerical Methods for Image Registration. Oxford University Press on Demand, Oxford (2004)

9. Pace, D.F., Aylward, S.R., Niethammer, M.: A locally adaptive regularization based on anisotropic diffusion for deformable image registration of sliding organs. IEEE Trans. Med. Imaging **32**(11), 2114–2126 (2013)
10. Papież, B.W., Heinrich, M.P., Fehrenbach, J., Risser, L., Schnabel, J.A.: An implicit sliding-motion preserving regularisation via bilateral filtering for deformable image registration. Med. Image Anal. **18**(8), 1299–1311 (2014)
11. Preston, J.S., Joshi, S., Whitaker, R.: Deformation estimation with automatic sliding boundary computation. In: Ourselin, S., Joskowicz, L., Sabuncu, M.R., Unal, G., Wells, W. (eds.) MICCAI 2016. LNCS, vol. 9902, pp. 72–80. Springer, Cham (2016). https://doi.org/10.1007/978-3-319-46726-9_9
12. Risser, L., Vialard, F.X., Baluwala, H.Y., Schnabel, J.A.: Piecewise-diffeomorphic image registration: application to the motion estimation between 3D CT lung images with sliding conditions. Med. Image Anal. **17**(2), 182–193 (2013)
13. Rueckert, D., Sonoda, L.I., Hayes, C., Hill, D.L., Leach, M.O., Hawkes, D.J.: Non-rigid registration using free-form deformations: application to breast MR images. IEEE Trans. Med. Imaging **18**(8), 712–721 (1999)
14. Schmidt-Richberg, A., Werner, R., Handels, H., Ehrhardt, J.: Estimation of slipping organ motion by registration with direction-dependent regularization. Med. Image Anal. **16**(1), 150–159 (2012)
15. von Siebenthal, M., Szekely, G., Gamper, U., Boesiger, P., Lomax, A., Cattin, P.: 4D MR imaging of respiratory organ motion and its variability. Phys. Med. Biol. **52**(6), 1547 (2007)
16. Sotiras, A., Davatzikos, C., Paragios, N.: Deformable medical image registration: a survey. IEEE Trans. Med. Imaging **32**(7), 1153–1190 (2013)
17. Sun, W., Niessen, W.J., van Stralen, M., Klein, S.: Simultaneous multiresolution strategies for nonrigid image registration. IEEE Trans. Image Process. **22**(12), 4905–4917 (2013)
18. Thirion, J.P.: Image matching as a diffusion process: an analogy with Maxwell's demons. Med. Image Anal. **2**(3), 243–260 (1998)
19. Van Stralen, M., Pluim, J.P.: Optimal discrete multi-resolution deformable image registration. In: Proceedings of the Sixth IEEE International Conference on Symposium on Biomedical Imaging: From Nano to Macro, pp. 947–950. IEEE Press (2009)
20. Vandemeulebroucke, J., Sarrut, D., Clarysse, P., et al.: The POPI-model, a point-validated pixel-based breathing thorax model. In: XVth International Conference on the Use of Computers in Radiation Therapy (ICCR), vol. 2, pp. 195–199 (2007)
21. Viergever, M.A., Maintz, J.A., Klein, S., Murphy, K., Staring, M., Pluim, J.P.: A survey of medical image registration-under review. Med. Image Anal. **33**, 140–144 (2016)
22. Vishnevskiy, V., Gass, T., Székely, G., Goksel, O.: Total variation regularization of displacements in parametric image registration. In: Yoshida, H., Näppi, J., Saini, S. (eds.) Abdominal Imaging. Computational and Clinical Applications. ABD-MICCAI 2014. Lecture Notes in Computer Science, vol. 8676. Springer, Cham (2014). https://doi.org/10.1007/978-3-319-13692-9_20

Statistical Motion Mask and Sliding Registration

Björn Eiben[1]($\boxtimes$), Elena H. Tran[1], Martin J. Menten[2], Uwe Oelfke[2],
David J. Hawkes[1], and Jamie R. McClelland[1]

[1] Centre for Medical Image Computing, University College London, London, UK
bjoern.eiben.10@ucl.ac.uk
[2] Joint Department of Physics, The Institute of Cancer Research
and The Royal Marsden NHS Foundation Trust, London, UK

Abstract. Accurate registration of images depicting respiratory motion, e.g. 4DCT or 4DMR, can be challenging due to sliding motion that occurs between the chest wall and organs within the pleural sac (lungs, mediastinum, liver). In this paper we propose a methodology that (1) segments one of the images to be registered (the source or floating/moving image) into two distinct regions by fitting a statistical motion mask, and (2) registers the image with a modified B-spline registration algorithm that can account for sliding motion between the regions. This registration requires the segmentation of the regions in the source image domain as a signed distance map. Two underlying transformations allow the regions to deform independently, while a constraint term based on the transformed distance maps penalises gaps and overlaps between the regions. Although implemented in a B-spline algorithm, the required modifications are not specific to the transformation type and thus can be applied to parametric and non-parametric frameworks alike. The registration accuracy is evaluated using the landmark registration error on the basis of the publicly available DIR-Lab dataset. The overall average landmark error after registration is 1.21 mm and the average gap and overlap volumes are 26.4 cm^3 and 34.5 cm^3 respectively. The fitted statistical motion masks are compared to previously proposed motion masks and the corresponding mean Dice coefficient is 0.96.

Keywords: Sliding motion · B-Spline registration
Statistical shape model · Motion mask

1 Introduction

Registration of images which contain anatomical regions that slide along each other is an ongoing research topic. The major challenge is that registration is an ill-posed problem and thus requires some regularisation which usually constrains the transformation to be smooth. This smoothness assumption however is not true across a sliding interface where discontinuities in the transformation are

S. Klein et al. (Eds.): WBIR 2018, LNCS 10883, pp. 13–23, 2018.
https://doi.org/10.1007/978-3-319-92258-4_2

present. A prominent example where sliding occurs is respiratory motion of the lung along the chest wall, facilitated by the pleural sac that encloses not only the lungs and heart, but also liver and further lower abdominal organs. As a result, registration of images of the thorax depicting respiratory motion is challenging.

Several registration methods for handling sliding motion have been proposed in the literature [1,5,7,10,13,14]. Most of these methods require a segmentation of the sliding regions either in the target image or in both target and source image. But for applications such as contour propagation in radiotherapy, it is preferable to segment the source image where the contours have been defined. Furthermore, for combined motion modelling and motion compensated image reconstruction from partial image data [8] it is essential to segment the source image as the target 'images' may be partial image data (e.g. individual slices, projections) which can be very challenging or impossible to accurately segment. Some methods do not require a prior segmentation in either image, but use a regularisation term that permits sliding motion [13]. While such methods are appealing, there is a possibility they may not correctly represent the sliding motion in areas of homogeneous intensities, for instance where the liver meets the chest wall. Furthermore, they do not model a true discontinuous motion, but approximate the sliding as a shear motion. However, it is acknowledged that while the discontinuous motion is more realistic, in practice this may not be important. Therefore, for some applications such as motion modelling from partial image data or radiotherapy dose accumulation, it may be desirable to explicitly specify where the sliding motion should occur, especially if parts of the sliding interface are not easily identifiable in the images. To the best of our knowledge, none of the published methods that require a segmentation allows the sliding regions to be specified only in the source image domain.

Identification of the sliding regions in CT images was proposed by Vandemeulebroucke et al. [12]. Their motion mask includes the lungs and other inferior organs that slide together and is thus anatomically more plausible than just a lung segmentation. However, this motion mask generation is designed specifically for CT images as it utilises features that can be relatively easily segmented from such images, namely lungs, thorax, and bones. Moreover, application of our implementation of this method proved to be time consuming because, (1) level-set evolutions are computationally expensive and (2) we did not find a single set of parameters that worked across all patients. Some manual corrections of the bony structures were also required where pacemakers or high intensity abdominal regions were present and morphologically connected to the bones.

The purpose of this paper is therefore twofold. In Sect. 2.1 we propose a motion mask generation on the basis of a statistical shape model [4] being fit to the source image. A resulting signed distance map where the zero-crossing identifies the interface of sliding image regions is then utilised by our sliding B-spline registration. The sliding framework is presented in Sect. 2.2. The results are quantitatively evaluated on the publicly available DIR-Lab dataset [2,3].

2   Materials and Methods

2.1   Statistical Motion Masks

The motion mask generation by Vandemeulebroucke et al. [12] uses a sequence of level-set evolutions that are controlled by three CT-based feature images, namely lungs, thorax, and bones. This method produces suitable motion masks from CT images, but cannot be used with MR images (which we intend to apply our method to in the future), and can be time consuming. Therefore, we build a statistical shape model of the motion masks from a large number of 4DCT images, that captures the inter-patient variation in the motion masks. This statistical shape model can then be used to segment a new image more rapidly than the original method, and can potentially be used on MR images. This shape model is fitted to directional intensity gradients which are present in both CT and MR images, such as the low-to-high intensity contrast between lung and surrounding tissue or the high-to-low contrast between thorax and air.

The generation of the statistical motion mask comprises of the following steps and is summarised in Fig. 1:

1. Calculate intra-subject average 4DCT image by group-wise registration,
2. Generate motion mask based on average 4DCT images according to [12],
3. Inter-patient group-wise registration of average 4DCT images,

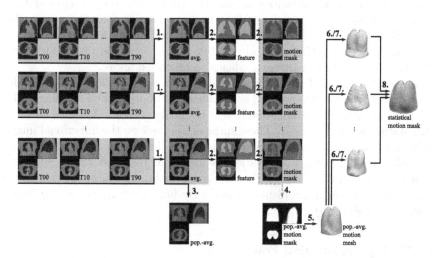

Fig. 1. Flow chart for the generation of the statistical motion mask. (1) Average 4DCT images (avg.) are generated by intra-patient group-wise registration of the different phases (T00-T90). (2) From these average images features are extracted and motion masks are calculated for each subject. (3) Inter-subject group-wise registration of average 4DCT images and (4) application of the transformations to the mask to create a population average motion mask. (5) A surface mesh is generated from the average motion mask image. (6/7) The surface mesh is transformed back to the individual images. (8) The deformations are captured in a statistical motion mask.

4. Use registration results to form the population-average motion mask image,
5. Convert population-average motion mask image into mesh representation,
6. Use registration results to transform motion mask mesh to each subject,
7. Refine mesh to better match individual motion mask images [6],
8. Statistical motion mask calculation [4].

A prerequisite for building a statistical shape model is the point-to-point correspondence between individual motion mask meshes (7) [4]. This is why one population-average motion mask mesh is generated (5) and then transformed back to each subject (6/7), rather than simply generating the meshes from each individual motion mask image. As the transformed mesh does not perfectly match the individual motion mask images due to registration errors, the mesh is refined by a surface alignment algorithm [6] where the transformed average mesh is iteratively deformed towards a target surface, in this case the motion masks calculated in (2). The final statistical shape model is formed by applying PCA on the refined mesh coordinates, and comprises the average shape and eigenvectors/principal components that define the modes of variation of the shape.

Once the statistical motion mask exists, an appearance representation in the form of intensity gradients is calculated along the mesh normals determining for each node if positive, negative or mixed intensity gradients dominate. Such gradients are measured in the direction of the outward facing mesh normals on the average 4DCT images. Only those nodes that have a clear positive or negative intensity gradient across all subjects will be used during mask fitting.

To fit the statistical motion mask to an image, i.e. finding the weights for each mode of variation and a global rigid transformation, we follow the iterative multi-scale process by Cootes et al. [4], but make the shape model lock onto either positive or negative image gradients as identified above.

Due to the shape of the motion mask, the positioning and extent in the inferior part of the mask is not well constrained. To improve the SI-scaling of the mask, we also include the lung-diaphragm boundary as two additional surfaces to the statistical motion mask. These surfaces also lock on the directional image gradients in the diaphragm region. This improves the scaling of the fitted mask in the SI-direction. For our application we also want the mask to extend below the image boundaries. Hence during the mask fitting the most inferior nodes of the statistical model are displaced inferiorly until they are below the image boundary (c.f. Fig. 4(b)).

2.2 Sliding Registration Framework

The proposed sliding framework uses two separate transformations for the two regions involved, region A and region B. This facilitates independent motion and thus the desired deformation discontinuity at the regions' interface. The corresponding transformations are denoted as $\mathbf{T}_A(\mathbf{x})$ and $\mathbf{T}_B(\mathbf{x})$. The method also requires a signed distance map $D(\mathbf{x})$ which defines the two regions, and can be pre-calculated based on the fitted statistical motion mask. Let region A be identified by negative values $D < 0$ and region B by positive values $D \geq 0$.

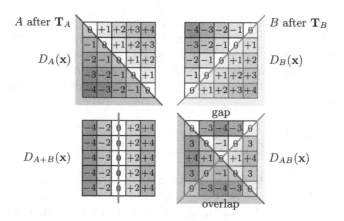

Fig. 2. Schematic of transformed distance maps D_A and D_B, their sum D_{A+B} and product D_{AB} as they are used in the sliding registration approach. The green overlay depicts region A after transformation with $\mathbf{T}_A$ and the yellow overlay shows region B after $\mathbf{T}_B$. The grey line (bottom left) indicates the boundary where the transformation switches from $\mathbf{T}_A$ to $\mathbf{T}_B$ and negative values of D_{AB} indicate gaps and overlaps. (Color figure online)

In order to calculate the deformed image it is necessary to determine which of the two transformations to use for each voxel in the target image. This is done by deforming the distance map with both transformations, $D_A(\mathbf{x}) = D(\mathbf{T}_A(\mathbf{x}))$ and $D_B(\mathbf{x}) = D(\mathbf{T}_B(\mathbf{x}))$, and summing the resulting deformed distance maps, $D_{A+B} = D_A + D_B$. Then

$$\mathbf{T}(\mathbf{x}) = \begin{cases} \mathbf{T}_A(\mathbf{x}) & \text{for } D_{A+B}(\mathbf{x}) < 0 \\ \mathbf{T}_B(\mathbf{x}) & \text{otherwise} \end{cases}. \tag{1}$$

The independent motion of the two regions can result in gaps between or overlap of the two regions. The above approach for determining which transformation should be used at each voxel means that the transition between using $\mathbf{T}_A$ and $\mathbf{T}_B$ will occur in the middle of any gaps and overlaps (see Fig. 2). However, even with this approach the gaps and overlaps will still lead to a violation of a one-to-one mapping between the images. Therefore, a gap-overlap constraint term (GOCT) is introduced, which is based on the product of the deformed distance maps $D_{AB} = D_A D_B$, and penalises any gaps and overlaps that occur (see Fig. 2). This term is non-zero only at positions where gaps and overlaps occur.

$$\mathcal{C}_{\text{GOCT}}(\mathbf{x}) = \begin{cases} -D_{AB}(\mathbf{x}) & \text{for } D_{AB}(\mathbf{x}) < 0 \\ 0 & \text{otherwise} \end{cases} \tag{2}$$

The total value of the constraint term is then calculated as the sum of $\mathcal{C}_{\text{GOCT}}$ over all voxels normalised by the number of voxels.

The transformations are both optimised simultaneously by calculating the gradient of the cost function (i.e. sum of similarity metric(s), $\mathcal{C}_{\text{GOCT}}$, and other constraint terms) with respect to each of the individual transformations. When calculating the gradient of the similarity metric(s) with respect to $\mathbf{T}_A$, only the voxels that are transformed by $\mathbf{T}_A$ (i.e. $D_{A+B} < 0$) contribute towards the gradient calculation. And likewise, only voxels transformed by $\mathbf{T}_B$ contribute towards the gradient with respect to $\mathbf{T}_B$. The gradient of $\mathcal{C}_{\mathrm{GOCT}}$ with respect to $\mathbf{T}_A$ is given by

$$\frac{\partial \mathcal{C}_{\mathrm{GOCT}}(\mathbf{x})}{\partial \mathbf{T}_A(\mathbf{x})} = \begin{cases} -D_B(\mathbf{x})\frac{\partial D_A(\mathbf{x})}{\partial T_A(\mathbf{x})} & \text{for } D_A(\mathbf{x})D_B(\mathbf{x}) < 0 \\ 0 & \text{otherwise} \end{cases}, \quad (3)$$

where $\partial D_A(\mathbf{x})/\partial T_A(\mathbf{x})$ is the spatial gradient of the distance map warped by the deformation field for region A. The gradients of any other constraint terms are calculated for each transformation separately, in exactly the same way as they would be for a standard (non-sliding) registration.

The sliding framework was used to modify NiftyReg, an open source B-spline registration software [9].

2.3   Image and Landmark Data

To build the statistical motion masks, 4DCT datasets from 32 subjects were used, each comprising of 10 respiratory phases. The first ten image sets were taken from the publicly available *DIR-Lab* dataset [2,3]. The remaining datasets were acquired as part of standard clinical practice from patients with either early-stage (14 cases) or locally-advanced (8 cases) non-small cell lung cancer.

The DIR-Lab dataset also contains 300 manually selected corresponding landmarks in the end-exhale and end-inhale phases. These were used to quantify the registration accuracy in terms of a landmark registration error (LME). Note that most of the LME values given on the DIR-Lab website have been calculated using the 'snap-to-voxel' approach [3], so for comparability reasons we also follow the same approach here.

3   Results

3.1   Statistical Motion Mask Fitting Accuracy

The fitting accuracy of the statistical motion mask with respect to the number of modes included in the model was evaluated against the level-set based motion mask in terms of the Dice coefficient and mean contour distance by using a leave-one-out evaluation strategy. To evaluate the dependency of the fitting accuracy on the number of modes of variation (i.e. number of eigenvectors of the statistical shape model), the fitting was performed in a multi-scale fashion with three resolution levels corresponding to intensity sampling distances along the mesh normal of 4 mm, 2 mm, and 1 mm and 200 iterations per level. The results are shown as box-plots in Fig. 3. The highest mean Dice coefficient of 0.96 ± 0.02 was achieved with 20 modes, whereas the lowest mean contour distance of 3.67 ± 2.00 mm was achieved with 25 modes.

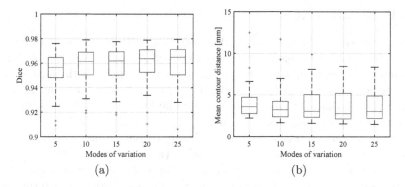

Fig. 3. Motion mask fitting accuracy in terms of the Dice coefficient (a) and mean contour distance (b). Red line represents the median value, the box extends from the first and the third quartile, and the whiskers extend the box by 1.5 times the interquartile range. (Color figure online)

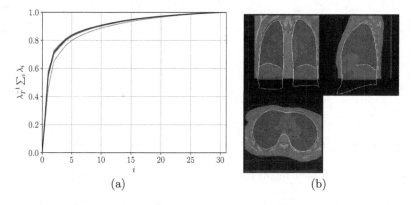

Fig. 4. (a) Cumulative, relative variation described by statistical shape model as a function of the number of modes of variation, i, used in the 32 leave-one-out models. For each model a grey curve is plotted and the average over all models is shown in black. (b) Level-set based motion mask (red) and statistical motion mask (white line) fitted to case 1 of the DIR-Lab dataset. (Color figure online)

Furthermore the variation covered by the shape model as a function of the number of modes is given in Fig. 4(a). For a coverage of 95% of the variation observed in the dataset 16 modes are required, and for 98% coverage 23 modes. After considering the Dice coefficient results, the mean contour distance results, and the percentage of variation covered, it was decided to use 23 modes for all the following experiments. An example result for this fitting configuration for the first case of the DIR-Lab dataset is shown in Fig. 4(b) along with the level-set based result.

3.2   Registration Accuracy

The registration accuracy was quantified using the DIR-Lab datasets as follows: The source image was selected to be the end-exhale image and the statistical motion mask (built leaving out the current dataset) was fitted in the same fashion as described in Sect. 3.1 using 23 modes of variation. A signed distance map was calculated from that motion mask and used as input into the sliding registration. In order to keep the number of parameters for the registration to a minimum, no other constraint terms were used. Different B-spline control point spacings ($s_x = [5, 10, \ldots, 30]$ mm) and $\mathcal{C}_{\text{GOCT}}$ weights ($w_{\text{go}} = [0.8, 0.85, 0.9, 0.95]$) were investigated. For comparison, standard, i.e. non-sliding, B-spline registrations with the same control-point spacings and no additional constraint terms were performed and evaluated. For all registrations Local Normalised Cross Correlation (LNCC) was used as the similarity measure.

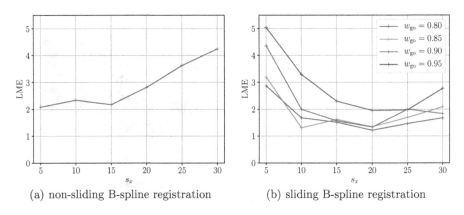

(a) non-sliding B-spline registration   (b) sliding B-spline registration

Fig. 5. Mean landmark errors (LME) over all 10 DIR-lab datasets and all landmarks after registration with respect to the control point spacing s_x. For the sliding registration results, (b), errors are given for several gap-overlap-constraint weights, w_{go}. All values are given in mm.

The landmark errors after alignment with the standard B-spline registration are shown in Fig. 5(a). Here the lowest average LME is 2.09 mm and results from a control-point spacing of $s_x = 5$ mm. The LME increases for coarser control-point grids.

The results for the sliding registration are shown in Fig. 5(b). The lowest average LME of 1.21 mm is achieved for a gap/overlap constraint weight $w_{\text{go}} = 0.8$ and a control-point spacing of $s_x = 20$ mm. However, results with this spacing and $w_{\text{go}} = [0.8, 0.85, 0.9]$ are very close together and below 1.34 mm. Compared with other methods, our resulting average landmark registration error is lower than those reported for instance by Papiez et al. [10] (1.95 mm), Wu et al. [14] (1.47 mm), Delmon et al. [5] (1.66 mm), and Berendsen et al. [1] (1.36 mm); but slightly larger the one reported by Hua et al. [7] (1.17 mm) or

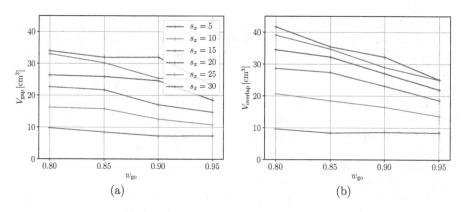

Fig. 6. Gap (a) and overlap (b) volumes in cubic centimetres with respect to the corresponding constraint weight w_{go} for several control point spacings s_x.

Table 1. Gap (V_{gap}) and overlap volumes ($V_{overlap}$) of segmentation-based methods as reported in the literature [1,5,7,14]. All values are given in cm^3.

	Wu 2008	Delmon 2013	Berendsen 2014	Hua 2017	Our method
V_{gap}	88.2	80.0	76.5	94.0	26.4
$V_{overlap}$	52.5	55.1	37.4	18.8	34.5
$V_{gap} \cup V_{overlap}$	130.7	135.1	113.9	112.8	60.9

Vishnevskiy et al. [13] (0.95 mm). A comprehensive list of landmark errors achieved by various algorithms is published on the DIR-Lab website [11].

Figure 6 shows the average gap and overlap volumes given in cubic centimetres as a function of the gap/overlap constraint weight for all tested control-point spacings. Gap and overlap volumes decrease towards higher constraint weights and smaller control point spacings. For the configuration that produces the lowest LME, the average gap and overlap volumes are 26.4 cm^3 and 34.5 cm^3 respectively. For comparison, gap, overlap and their combined volumes as reported by [1,5,7,14] for segmentation-based methods on the same DIR-Lab dataset are shown in Table 1.

4   Discussion and Conclusion

In this paper we present a method to register images which contain regions that slide along each other, and demonstrating this on 4DCTs of the thorax. To achieve this source images are segmented into sliding regions by fitting a statistical motion mask which encompasses the lungs, heart and further inferior organs. This segmentation is used as an additional input for a modified B-spline registration. The modification implements a sliding framework that allows for using different transformation types and/or other constraint terms for each region.

Defining the sliding regions in the source image domain can be beneficial for applications such as contour propagation for radiotherapy, and is required for motion modelling, and motion compensated image reconstruction from partial image data [8].

The statistical motion mask fitting is an extension of the work of Vandemeulebroucke et al. [12] who calculate a motion mask on the basis of image features that are extracted from CT images and multiple level-set evolution steps. This procedure is computationally expensive and is only applicable to CT images. The statistical motion mask can be fitted relatively fast and the method is designed to be applicable to MR as well as CT images. However, a quantitative evaluation on MR images will be subject of future work.

The sliding registration requires the segmentation of the two regions in the form of a signed distance map that can be pre-calculated. Each region is associated with a separate transformation which allows the regions to move independently from each other. A new constraint term has been used to help prevent gaps and overlaps occurring between the two regions, and hence maintain a one-to-one mapping between the images.

The proposed registration method achieved an average registration accuracy of 1.21 mm. These errors are based on manually identified correspondences and thus are subject to inter- and intra-observer errors which range between 0.70 mm and 1.13 mm [2]. This poses a lower limit on the measurable accuracy. While the DIR-Lab dataset provides an excellent tool for algorithm comparison, tests of statistical significance of algorithm performances however are not possible without gaining access to the full landmark error distributions for all algorithms being compared. Furthermore our method outperformed other segmentation based methods in terms of combined gap and overlap volumes. The reduction in gap and overlap volumes could be important for applications such as radiotherapy dose accumulation, but further work is required to demonstrate this.

One limitation of our method is that currently only two regions can be handled. Nevertheless, from our experiments this is sufficient for registrations of the respiratory motion in the thorax.

Acknowledgements. This research is funded by the Stand Up to Cancer campaign for Cancer Research UK (C33589/A19727, C33589/A19908, C33589/CRC521) and Network Accelerator Award Grant (A219932). We acknowledge financial and technical support from Elekta AB under a research agreement and NHS funding to the NIHR Biomedical Research Centre at RMH/ICR.

References

1. Berendsen, F.F., Kotte, A.N.T.J., Viergever, M.A., Pluim, J.P.W.: Registration of organs with sliding interfaces and changing topologies. In: Proceedings of SPIE Medical Imaging, vol. 9034, pp. 1–7 (2014)
2. Castillo, E., Castillo, R., Martinez, J., Shenoy, M., Guerrero, T.: Four-dimensional deformable image registration using trajectory modeling. Phys. Med. Biol. **55**(1), 305–327 (2010)

3. Castillo, R., Castillo, E., Guerra, R., Johnson, V.E., McPhail, T., Garg, A.K., Guerrero, T.: A framework for evaluation of deformable image registration spatial accuracy using large landmark point sets. Phys. Med. Biol. **54**(7), 1849–1870 (2009)
4. Cootes, T.F., Taylor, C.J., et al.: Statistical models of appearance for computer vision. Technical report, University of Manchester (2004)
5. Delmon, V., Rit, S., Pinho, R., Sarrut, D.: Registration of sliding objects using direction dependent B-splines decomposition. Phys. Med. Biol. **58**(5), 1303–1314 (2013)
6. Eiben, B., Vavourakis, V., Hipwell, J.H., Kabus, S., Lorenz, C., Buelow, T., Williams, N.R., Keshtgar, M., Hawkes, D.J.: Surface driven biomechanical breast image registration. In: Proceedings of SPIE Medical Imaging, vol. 9786, pp. 1–10 (2016)
7. Hua, R., Pozo, J.M., Taylor, Z.A., Frangi, A.F.: Multiresolution eXtended Free-Form Deformations (XFFD) for non-rigid registration with discontinuous transforms. Med. Image Anal. **36**, 113–122 (2017)
8. McClelland, J.R., Modat, M., Arridge, S., Grimes, H., D'Souza, D., Thomas, D., Connell, D.O., Low, D.A., Kaza, E., Collins, D.J., Leach, M.O., Hawkes, D.J.: A generalized framework unifying image registration and respiratory motion models and incorporating image reconstruction, for partial image data or full images. Phys. Med. Biol. **62**(11), 4273–4292 (2017)
9. Modat, M., Ridgway, G.R., Taylor, Z.A., Lehmann, M., Barnes, J., Hawkes, D.J., Fox, N.C., Ourselin, S.: Fast free-form deformation using graphics processing units. Comput. Methods Programs Biomed. **98**(3), 278–284 (2010)
10. Papiez, B.W., Heinrich, M.P., Fehrenbach, J., Risser, L., Schnabel, J.A.: An implicit sliding-motion preserving regularisation via bilateral filtering for deformable image registration. Med. Image Anal. **18**(8, SI), 1299–1311 (2014)
11. The Deformable Image Registration Laboratory: DIR Spatial Accuracy Results (2018). https://www.dir-lab.com/Results.html. Accessed 20 Mar 2018
12. Vandemeulebroucke, J., Bernard, O., Rit, S., Kybic, J., Clarysse, P., Sarrut, D.: Automated segmentation of a motion mask to preserve sliding motion in deformable registration of thoracic CT. Med. Phys. **39**, 1006–1015 (2012)
13. Vishnevskiy, V., Gass, T., Szekely, G., Tanner, C., Goksel, O.: Isotropic total variation regularization of displacements in parametric image registration. IEEE Trans. Med. Imaging **36**(2), 385–395 (2017)
14. Wu, Z., Rietzel, E., Boldea, V., Sarrut, D., Sharp, G.C.: Evaluation of deformable registration of patient lung 4DCTs with subanatomical region segmentations. Med. Phys. **35**(2), 775–781 (2008)

Adaptive Graph Diffusion Regularisation for Discontinuity Preserving Image Registration

Robin Sandkühler[✉], Christoph Jud, Simon Pezold, and Philippe C. Cattin

Department of Biomedical Engineering, University of Basel, Allschwil, Switzerland
robin.sandkuehler@unibas.ch

Abstract. Registration of thoracic images is central when studying for example physiological changes of the lung. Due to sliding organ motion and intensity changes based on respiration the registration of thoracic images is challenging. We present a novel regularisation method based on adaptive anisotropic graph diffusion. Without the need of a mask it preserves discontinuities of the transformation at sliding organ boundaries and enforces smoothness in areas with similar motion. The graph diffusion regularisation provides a direct way to achieve anisotropic diffusion at sliding organ boundaries by reducing the weight of corresponding edges in the graph which cross the sliding interfaces. Since the graph diffusion is defined by the edge weights of the graph, we develop an adaptive edge weight function to detect sliding boundaries. We implement the adaptive graph diffusion regularisation method in the Demons registration framework. The presented method is tested on synthetic 2D images and on the public 4D-CT DIR-Lab data set, where we are able to correctly detect the sliding organ boundaries.

1 Introduction

The registration of images of the human thorax is essential for the analysis or the monitoring of physiological properties of the upper abdomen. However, thoracic images are affected by sliding organ motion at the thoracic cavity, and corresponding mass points undergo cyclic intensity changes over the respiratory cycle. If images are affected by sliding organ motion the global smoothness assumption of the transformation often does not hold, because of local discontinuities in the transformation at these boundaries.

Several registration approaches haven been presented to overcome the trade-off between global smoothness and local discontinuity preservation. Based on their definition parametric approaches are more likely to achieve global smoothness, if the chosen basis function is smooth. In order to preserve local discontinuities with a parametric approach, a stationary first order B-spline kernel combined with a Total Variation (TV) regularisation is introduced in [19]. A non-stationary kernel is described in [6]. Here, a smooth kernel is locally adapted in its shape based on the image intensities. Non-parametric approaches are well suited

© Springer International Publishing AG, part of Springer Nature 2018
S. Klein et al. (Eds.): WBIR 2018, LNCS 10883, pp. 24–34, 2018.
https://doi.org/10.1007/978-3-319-92258-4_3

for local discontinuity preservation, as they directly estimate the transformation for each pixel. Different direction-dependent regularisation methods based on the image intensities or the transformation are presented in [4,11,16]. In [12] an adaptive Gaussian regularisation based on bilateral filtering is shown. Segmentation of the sliding boundaries can also be used by either building a motion segmentation [7] during the registration, or assuming a prior segmentation to locally adapt the transformation model [5]. Several graph based approaches have been introduced in the past. Using a graph based formulation for TV regularisation [2] or a non-local regularisation based on the minimum spanning tree of a graph [13]. In both methods the image intensities are used to calculate the edge weights of the graph.

As mentioned before parametric approaches are well suited for global smoothness, and non-parametric regularisation, especially anisotropic diffusion [4,11,16], are effective to preserve local discontinuities. In order to achieve both, we propose the graph diffusion as regularisation method for image registration. Graph diffusion allows global smoothness while at the same time local differences on the pixel level are considered. It was shown to be a valid regularisation operator for kernel-based learning algorithms [17] and a reliable and computationally efficient method in the area of edge-preserving image smoothing [20]. Anisotropic diffusion can be achieved with graph diffusion in a straightforward way by modifying the edge weight between nodes. In order to achieve anisotropic diffusion at local discontinuities, we need to reduce the edge weights of nodes which are located on different sites of a sliding organ boundary.

In this work, we present the adaptive anisotropic graph diffusion regularisation method (A^2GD) to enforce global smoothness and preserve local discontinuities of the transformation. We achieve this without prior information (e.g. segmentation) of the sliding organ boundaries. A local adaptive edge weight function is developed to create anisotropic diffusion only at sliding organ interfaces and isotropic diffusion in areas with similar motion. The proposed regularisation is implemented in the Demons framework [18] and replaces the isotropic diffusion regularisation. To the extent of our knowledge, graph diffusion has not been used as regularisation method for image registration before.

2   Background

Let $T, R : \mathcal{X} \to \mathbb{R}$ be the target and reference image over the image domain $\mathcal{X}$. We define the image domain $\mathcal{X} = \{x_i\}_{i=1}^n$ as a set of regular distributed grid points x_i in d-dimensions. The registration problem can be defined as a regularised minimisation problem:

$$f = \arg\min_u \mathcal{S}[T, R_u] + \varphi\mathcal{R}[u], \tag{1}$$

where transformation of interest $f : \mathcal{X} \to \mathbb{R}^d$ is a minimiser of (1). Here, $\mathcal{S}[\cdot, \cdot]$ is the similarity measure for the target image T and the transformed reference image R_f with $R_f(x_i) = R(x_i + f(x_i))$. In order to restrict the space of admissible transformations, prior knowledge of the transformation space (e.g. smoothness) can be applied to the registration problem by the regularisation term $\mathcal{R}[\cdot]$. The parameter φ controls the influence of the regularisation e.g. the smoothness of the transformation. A possible method to find a transformation that minimises (1) is the Demons method proposed by Thirion [18]. He proposed an iterative method to determine f by alternating minimising the similarity $\mathcal{S}$ and computing the regularisation $\mathcal{R}$. A generalisation of this idea is shown in Algorithm 1. Thirion proposed an isotropic diffusion process as regularisation to smooth the transformation. Isotropic diffusion can be achieved by

$$\mathcal{R}_{\mathrm{ID}}[f] = K_\varphi^{\mathrm{G}} * f^l \quad l = 1, \dots, d \tag{2}$$

for each spatial dimension l. Here, $*$ is the convolution and K_φ^{G} is a Gaussian kernel (diffusion kernel) with a kernel size of $\sqrt{2\varphi}$ [1].

Algorithm 1. Demons registration framework

1: **Inputs:**
    T, R, $N :=$ number of iterations, $\sigma :=$ kernel size, $\alpha :=$ step size
2: **Initialise:**
    $f \leftarrow 0$
3: **for** i $= 1$ to N **do**
4:     $s \leftarrow \nabla S[T, R_f]$ compute image force (demons)
5:     $f \leftarrow f + \alpha s$ update transformation
6:     $f \leftarrow K_\sigma * f$ smooth transformation

---

3   Method

We summarise in the following the definition of diffusion on graphs, how it can be calculated efficiently, and how we use it as regularisation for image registration. Further, we propose our extension the adaptive anisotropic graph diffusion regulariser ($\mathrm{A}^2\mathrm{GD}$), and an edge weight function to detect sliding organ boundaries.

3.1   Adaptive Graph Diffusion Regularisation

In order to apply graph diffusion as regularisation $\mathcal{R}_{\mathrm{GD}}[f]$, the transformation f is modelled as an undirected weighted grid graph $\mathcal{G} = (V, E, W)$ with n nodes. Each node $v_i \in V$, with the node position $x_i \in \mathcal{X}$, represents $f(x_i)$. The set of edges is given as $E \subseteq V \times V$. An edge $e_{ij} \in E$ connects the nodes v_i and v_j. The weight matrix $W \in \mathbb{R}^{n \times n}$ contains the edge weights of the graph with $W(i, j) = w(e_{ij})$ and $w : E \to [0, 1]$. A central element in spectral graph theory is the graph Laplacian matrix $L \in \mathbb{R}^{n \times n}$. The Laplacian matrix is a symmetric matrix and is defined as $L = D - W$ with

$$L(i, j) = \begin{cases} D(i, j) - W(i, j), & \text{if } i = j \\ -W(i, j), & \text{if } e_{ij} \in E \\ 0, & \text{otherwise,} \end{cases} \tag{3}$$

where $D \in \mathbb{R}^{n \times n}$ is the diagonal degree matrix with $D(i, i) = \sum_{j=1}^{n} W(i, j)$.

The diffusion rate or the flow between two nodes is determined by the weight of the edge between both nodes. This allows to define arbitrary anisotropic diffusion by only modifying the edge weights of the graph. In order to define the diffusion process on graphs, Eq. (2) can be rewritten as

$$\mathcal{R}_{\mathrm{GD}}[f] = K_{\varphi}^{\mathrm{GD}} \bar{f}^l = \exp(-\varphi L)\bar{f}^l \quad l = 1, \ldots, d. \tag{4}$$

Here, $\bar{f}^i \in \mathbb{R}^{n \times 1}$ is the column vector representation of the transformation f and $K_{\varphi}^{\mathrm{GD}} \in \mathbb{R}^{n \times n}$ is the graph diffusion kernel [8,20] with the matrix exponential $\exp(\cdot)$. If the edge weights are set according to the node position x_i and x_j with $w(e_{ij}) = \exp(-||x_i - x_j||^2/4\varphi)$, then (2) and (4) will provide the same results. We refer the reader to [20] for a more detailed description of graph diffusion.

In order to achieve an adaptive graph diffusion regularisation we make the graph diffusion kernel $K_{\varphi}^{\mathrm{GD}}$ non-static. We do this by updating the edge weights in the weight matrix W_k in each iteration k with the edge weight function presented bellow. The final adaptive graph diffusion regularisation is defined as

$$\mathcal{R}_{A^2GD}[f_{k+1}, W_k] = K_{\varphi}^{\mathrm{GD}}(W_k)\bar{f}^l_{k+1} = \exp(-\varphi L(W_k))\bar{f}^l_{k+1} \quad l = 1, \ldots, d. \tag{5}$$

Computation of the Graph Diffusion. Calculating the matrix exponential of the Laplace matrix L is the major computational challenge for the graph diffusion. For the matrix L, the matrix exponential can be defined as

$$\exp(L) = \sum_{k=0}^{\infty} \frac{1}{k!} L^k. \tag{6}$$

Different approaches exists to compute the matrix exponential [10]. The graph Laplacian matrix L can be of high order, therefore the computation becomes costly. However, the explicit calculation of the matrix exponential is not required for the graph diffusion. In order to compute the graph diffusion only the action of the graph diffusion kernel to the transformation vector is needed (4). It has been shown in [14] that those kind of actions can be efficiently approximated with the Krylov subspace projection methods. Therefore, $\exp(L)f$ is approximated by an element of the Krylov subspace $K_m(L, f) = \mathrm{span}\{f, Lf, L^2f, \ldots, L^{m-1}f\}$, where m is the dimension of the Krylov subspace. Normally the Krylov space dimension ($m < 50$) is much smaller compared to n which can be in the range of a few million in case of 3D registration. Since L is a hermitian matrix, the Lanczos algorithm [9] offers a computationally efficient way to find the approximating element of $K_m(L, f)$. The final approximation of (4) is then given as

$$\bar{f}^l_{\mathrm{smooth}} = \exp(-\varphi L)\bar{f}^l \approx ||\bar{f}^l||_2 P \exp(Q)e_1. \tag{7}$$

Here, $P \in \mathbb{R}^{n \times m}$ is the projection matrix, $Q \in \mathbb{R}^{m \times m}$ a symmetric tridiagonal matrix, and e_1 is the first unit vector. Both matrices P and Q are the results of the Lanczos algorithm. The approximation only requires the matrix exponential of a matrix with the order of m instead of the order of n. Since Q is a symmetric tridiagonal matrix, we compute the matrix exponential of Q by $\exp(Q) = \Lambda \exp(\Gamma)\Lambda^{-1}$. Each column in Λ is an eigenvector of Q and Γ is a diagonal matrix of the corresponding eigenvalues. The matrix exponential of Γ is the exponential of each diagonal element of Γ.

Local Edge Update. The graph diffusion allows an anisotropic diffusion process by modifying corresponding edge weights. However, detecting the corresponding edges only in one information domain (e.g. image intensities) is challenging, since sliding organ boundaries not always correspond to intensity differences (see Fig. 1, Case (I)). We define five cases (see Fig. 1) to adapt the edge weights either for anisotropic or isotropic diffusion. In Case (I) and (II), the edges crosses a sliding organ boundary and therefore their edge weights need to be zero to enforce anisotropic diffusion. The other edges are either inside the same organ (Case (III) and (V)) or crossing an organ boundary where both organs move similarly (Case (IV)). In cases (III) to (V) isotropic diffusion is desired and therefore the edge weights should be one. We propose a locally adaptive edge weight function to cover all five cases based on three different information domains. The first two are the image intensity domain (Case III, V)

$$w_{\mathrm{img}}(e_{ij}) = \exp(-\delta_{\mathrm{img}}\|T(x_i) - T(x_j)\|), \tag{8}$$

and the transformation domain (Case I–V)

$$w_{\mathrm{f}}(e_{ij}) = \exp(-\delta_{\mathrm{f}}\|f(x_i) - f(x_j)\|), \tag{9}$$

with the scaling parameter δ_{img} and δ_{f} The third domain is described by the relation between the direction of the image gradient and the direction of the transformation (Case II, IV) based on the Nagel-Enkelmann operator [11]. Adapting the pixel-wise Nagel-Enkelmann operator to an edge weight function for the graph diffusion results in

$$w_{\perp}(e_{ij}) = 0.5 \left(\frac{\|\nabla I_{\max}(e_{ij})f(x_i)^T\|}{\|\nabla I_{\max}(e_{ij})\|\,\|f(x_i)\|} + \frac{\|\nabla I_{\max}(e_{ij})f(x_j)^T\|}{\|\nabla I_{\max}(e_{ij})\|\,\|f(x_j)\|} \right) \tag{10}$$

with

$$\nabla I_{\max}(e_{i,j}) = \begin{cases} \nabla T(x_i), & \|\nabla T(x_i)\| \geq \|\nabla T(x_j)\| \\ \nabla T(x_j), & \text{otherwise.} \end{cases} \tag{11}$$

The final weight function is then given as

$$w(e_{ij}) = \tau w_{\mathrm{f}}(e_{ij}) + (1 - \tau)[(w_{\mathrm{img}}(e_{ij})w_{\mathrm{f}}(e_{ij}) + (1 - w_{\mathrm{img}})w_{\perp}(e_{ij})]. \tag{12}$$

The scale function $\tau \in [0, 1]$ in (12) allows to adapt the scale between the image based domains (8) and (10) and the transformation domain (9). The final edge weights are thresholded with

$$\bar{w}_k(e_{ij}) = \begin{cases} 0, & w_k(e_{ij}) < 0.5 \\ 1, & \text{else} \end{cases}. \tag{13}$$

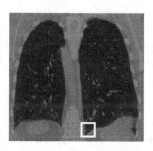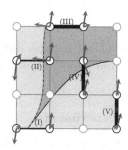

Fig. 1. Different cases, which are considered for the edge weight adaptation at sliding interfaces (dashed green) based on image gradients (red), transformation (blue) and intensity differences (gray values). (Color figure online)

In order to reduce the effect of oscillating edge weights an exponential smoothing

$$W_{k+1}(i,j) = \rho\, W_k(i,j) + (1 - \rho)\bar{w}_{k+1}(e_{ij}) \tag{14}$$

is applied, where ρ is the exponential decay rate.

Node Isolation. A node v_i is isolated from the graph, if all edges connected to this node have a zero weight $D(i,i) = 0$. Isolated nodes can cause artefacts in the transformation, because they are excluded from the regularisation. In order to prevent node isolation, all weights of the edges connected to a node v_i with $D(i,i) < \beta$ will be set to one. We choose $\beta \leq 2$ in 2D and $\beta \leq 3$ in 3D , so that the reset will not affect nodes at sliding boundaries.

3.2   Transformation Update

The update of the transformation in the Demons framework can be written in the form of a gradient descent update

$$f_{k+1} = f_k + \eta_k \nabla \mathcal{S}[T, R_{f_k}]. \tag{15}$$

In order to improve the convergence of the Demons framework we replace (15) by the well known Momentum optimiser equations

$$b_{k+1} = \alpha_k v_k + \eta_k \nabla \mathcal{S}[T, R_{f_k}] \tag{16}$$
$$f_{k+1} = f_k + b_{k+1} \tag{17}$$

as introduced in [15]. We set $\eta_k = 1/(\|\nabla R_{f_k}\|^2 + \psi)$ according to [18].

4   Results

We evaluated our adaptive graph diffusion regularisation method on synthetic 2D images with given ground truth, and on the public available DIR-Lab data sets.

4.1   Synthetic Experiments

We define a target image T with a size of 256×256 pixels and the intensities $T(x) = x \times e_1/\pi$, where e_1 is a unit vector (Fig. 2a). The inner part of the target image is rotated by $15°$ and the outer part is rotated in the opposite direction, in order to simulate a sliding boundary (Fig. 2b).

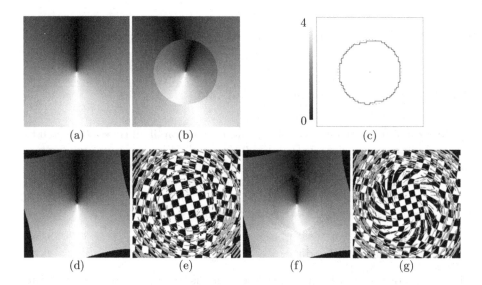

Fig. 2. Target image (a) and reference image (b) for the synthetic experiment. The red circle shows the sliding organ boundary between the inner and the outer region. Registration result with edge update (d) and the corresponding warped checker board (e), and without edge update (f) and the corresponding warped checker board (g). The graph degree matrix at the end of the registration is shown in (c).

The $\mathcal{S}_{\mathrm{MSE}}[T, R_f] = 1/n \sum_{i=1}^{n}(T(x_i) - R_f(x))^2$ metric is used as similarity measure. We choose $w(e_{ij}) = 0.5 \cdot (1 + ||f(x_i)^T f(x_j)||_2/||f(x_i)||_2||f(x_j)||_2)$ as edge weight function, because the sliding organ boundary in the image can be mainly described by direction differences of the displacement. Further, we used a multi-scale approach with three resolutions $\{64, 128, 256\}$. The regularisation parameter are set to $\varphi_0 = \{4, 8, 13\}$ and $\varphi_{\min} = \{1, 2, 2\}$. In each iteration the current regularisation weight is given by $\varphi_k = \varphi_0 * \exp(-0.05k) + \varphi_{\min}$ All remaining parameters are set as follows: $m = 30$, $\psi = 0.01$, $\rho = 0.9$, $\alpha = 0.9$, and $N = \{100, 100, 200\}$ iterations. All edge weights $w(e_{ij})$ are initialised with one.

The results of the proposed regularisation method for the synthetic experiments are shown in Fig. 2d with edge update and in Fig. 2f without edge update. With edge updates during the registration the ground truth displacement is very well estimated. The sliding boundary is clearly detected as we can see a reduction of the degree matrix values only at the sliding organ boundary (Fig. 2c). If we apply the transformation result from the method without the edge update to a checker board, we get strong distortion at the sliding boundary (Fig. 2g). Compared to this, our presented method reduce the distortion at sliding organ boundaries to a minimum (Fig. 2e).

4.2   DIR-Lab Data Set

The publicly available DIR-Lab[1] data set contains 10 4D-CT image series of different individuals. All images have a size between $256 \times 256 \times 94$ voxel and $512 \times 512 \times 136$ voxel, with a voxel size in the range of $0.97 \times 0.97 \times 2.5 \, \mathrm{mm}^3$ and $1.16 \times 1.16 \times 2.5 \, \mathrm{mm}^3$. For all images we clip the intensities between $50 \, \mathrm{HU}$ and $1200 \, \mathrm{HU}$, scale them in a range of $[0, 1]$, and resample all to a voxel size of $1 \times 1 \times 1 \, \mathrm{mm}^3$. For the evaluation of the registration result, the DIR-Lab data set provides 300 landmarks for the maximal inhalation and maximal exhalation of the breathing cycle. As images similarity measure the normalised local cross correlation $\mathcal{S}_{\mathrm{lcc}}$ is used. We use the derivative approximation of $\mathcal{S}_{\mathrm{lcc}}$ introduced in [3].

Table 1. Mean snap to voxel TRE in millimetre based on the 300 landmarks of DIR-Lab data set.

Case	#1	#2	#3	#4	#5	#6	#7	#8	#9	#10	Mean
No Reg	3.87	4.34	6.96	9.86	7.51	10.93	11.03	15.01	7.94	7.33	8.48
MST [13]	**0.83**	**0.87**	**1.10**	1.96	**1.36**	1.77	1.58	2.08	1.50	1.40	1.44
A^{2}GD	1.12	1.20	1.27	**1.61**	1.53	**1.32**	**1.38**	**1.45**	**1.36**	**1.34**	**1.36**

A multi-scale approach with four scales is used for the registration. At the end of each scale level, the transformation result is projected to the next scale level as initial value. All parameters are set as follows: $N = \{200, 200, 200, 300\}$, $m = 30$, $\rho = \{0.9\}$, $\sigma_{\mathrm{lcc}} = \{2, 8, 10, 15\}$, $\delta_{\mathrm{img}} = 5$, $\delta_{\mathrm{f}} = \{1, 0.5, 0.25, 0.125\}$, $\psi = \{0.5, 0.3, 0.2, 0.2\}$ and increased with 10^{-3}, The regularisation parameter is set to $\varphi = \{2, 3, 3, 3\}$. We set $\tau_0 = 0$ and increase it linear with a factor of 10^{-5} in each iteration. With this configuration the average run time is 5 min for one image pair on a GPU.

In Table 1 the mean TRE for all 10 data sets based on the 300 landmarks is shown. We compare our method to the MST based graph regularisation method [13]. As shown in Fig. 3 our method is able achieve global smoothness of the transformation and preserves discontinuities at sliding organ boundaries.

---

[1] http://www.dir-lab.com.

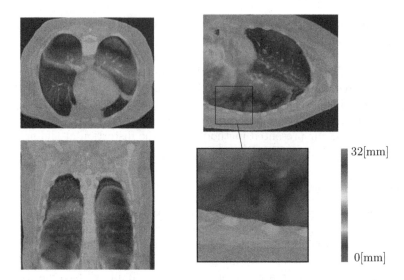

Fig. 3. Displacement field of the #8 case of the DIR-Lab data set.

5   Conclusion

We presented a novel regularisation method based on adaptive anisotropic graph diffusion. Without the need of a prior segmentation of the sliding organ boundaries our proposed regularisation method enforces global smoothness and preserves local discontinuities. In order to achieve anisotropic diffusion at sliding organ boundaries we developed an adaptive edge weight function based on local image intensities and the transformation. The results show that we are able to well detect the sliding organ boundaries and preserve the discontinuities in the transformation for the synthetic examples and for the DIR-Lab data set. We achieve a sub-millimetre difference, if we compare our TRE results to results of state of the art methods.

Acknowledgement. The authors would like to thank the Swiss National Science Foundation for funding this project (SNF 320030_149576).

References

1. Babaud, J., Witkin, A.P., Baudin, M., Duda, R.O.: Uniqueness of the Gaussian kernel for scale-space filtering. IEEE Trans. Pattern Anal. Mach. Intell. PAMI **8**(1), 26–33 (1986)
2. Bagnato, L., Frossard, P., Vandergheynst, P.: Optical flow and depth from motion for omnidirectional images using a TV-L1 variational framework on graphs. In: 2009 16th IEEE International Conference on Image Processing, pp. 1469–1472 (2009)

3. Cachier, P., Pennec, X.: 3D non-rigid registration by gradient descent on a Gaussian-windowed similarity measure using convolutions. In: Proceedings IEEE Workshop on Mathematical Methods in Biomedical Image Analysis, pp. 182–189 (2000)

4. Demirovic, D., Serifovic, A., Cattin, P.C.: An anisotropic diffusion regularized demons for improved registration of sliding organs. In: 18th International Electrotechnical and Computer Science Conference (ERK), p. BM.1.4 (2009)

5. Hua, R., Pozo, J.M., Taylor, Z.A., Frangi, A.F.: Multiresolution eXtended Free-Form Deformations (XFFD) for non-rigid registration with discontinuous transforms. Med. Image Anal. **36**, 113–122 (2017)

6. Jud, C., Möri, N., Bitterli, B., Cattin, P.C.: Bilateral regularization in reproducing kernel hilbert spaces for discontinuity preserving image registration. In: Wang, L., Adeli, E., Wang, Q., Shi, Y., Suk, H.-I. (eds.) MLMI 2016. LNCS, vol. 10019, pp. 10–17. Springer, Cham (2016). https://doi.org/10.1007/978-3-319-47157-0_2

7. Kiriyanthan, S., Fundana, K., Majeed, T., Cattin, P.C.: A primal-dual approach for discontinuity preserving image registration through motion segmentation. Int. J. Comput. Math. Methods Med. (2016)

8. Kondor, R.I., Lafferty, J.D.: Diffusion kernels on graphs and other discrete input spaces. In: Proceedings of the Nineteenth International Conference on Machine Learning, pp. 315–322. Morgan Kaufmann Publishers Inc., San Francisco (2002)

9. Lanczos, C.: An iteration method for the solution of the eigenvalue problem of linear differential and integral operators. J. Res. Natl. Bur. Stand. B **45**, 255–282 (1950)

10. Moler, C., Loan, C.V.: Nineteen dubious ways to compute the exponential of a matrix, twenty-five years later. SIAM Rev. **45**(1), 801–836 (2003)

11. Nagel, H.H., Enkelmann, W.: An investigation of smoothness constraints for the estimation of displacement vector fields from image sequences. IEEE Trans. Pattern Anal. Mach. Intell. PAMI **8**(5), 565–593 (1986)

12. Papież, B.W., Heinrich, M.P., Fehrenbach, J., Risser, L., Schnabel, J.A.: An implicit sliding-motion preserving regularisation via bilateral filtering for deformable image registration. Med. Image Anal. **18**(8), 1299–1311 (2014)

13. Papież, B.W., Szmul, A., Grau, V., Brady, J.M., Schnabel, J.A.: Non-local Graph-based regularization for deformable image registration. In: Müller, H., et al. (eds.) MCV/BAMBI -2016. LNCS, vol. 10081, pp. 199–207. Springer, Cham (2017). https://doi.org/10.1007/978-3-319-61188-4_18

14. Saad, Y.: Analysis of some Krylov subspace approximations to the matrix exponential operator. SIAM J. Numer. Anal. **29**(1), 209–228 (1992)

15. Santos-Ribeiro, A., Nutt, D.J., McGonigle, J.: Inertial demons: a momentum-based diffeomorphic registration framework. In: Ourselin, S., Joskowicz, L., Sabuncu, M.R., Unal, G., Wells, W. (eds.) MICCAI 2016. LNCS, vol. 9902, pp. 37–45. Springer, Cham (2016). https://doi.org/10.1007/978-3-319-46726-9_5

16. Schmidt-Richberg, A., Werner, R., Handels, H., Ehrhardt, J.: Estimation of slipping organ motion by registration with direction-dependent regularization. Med. Image Anal. **16**(1), 150–159 (2012)

17. Smola, A.J., Kondor, R.: Kernels and regularization on graphs. In: Schölkopf, B., Warmuth, M.K. (eds.) COLT-Kernel 2003. LNCS (LNAI), vol. 2777, pp. 144–158. Springer, Heidelberg (2003). https://doi.org/10.1007/978-3-540-45167-9_12

18. Thirion, J.P.: Image matching as a diffusion process: an analogy with Maxwell's demons. Med. Image Anal. **2**, 243–260 (1998)

19. Vishnevskiy, V., Gass, T., Szekely, G., Tanner, C., Goksel, O.: Isotropic total variation regularization of displacements in parametric image registration. IEEE Trans. Med. Imaging **36**(2), 385–395 (2017)
20. Zhang, F., Hancock, E.R.: Graph spectral image smoothing using the heat kernel. Pattern Recognit. **41**(11), 3328–3342 (2008)

Groupwise Registration

Fast Groupwise 4D Deformable Image Registration for Irregular Breathing Motion Estimation

Bartłomiej W. Papież[1,2(✉)], Daniel R. McGowan[3,4], Michael Skwarski[3], Geoff S. Higgins[3], Julia A. Schnabel[2,5], and Sir Michael Brady[3]

[1] Big Data Institute, Li Ka Shing Centre for Health Information and Discovery, University of Oxford, Oxford, UK

[2] Institute of Biomedical Engineering, Department of Engineering Science, University of Oxford, Oxford, UK
`bartlomiej.papiez@eng.ox.ac.uk`

[3] Department of Oncology, University of Oxford, Oxford, UK

[4] Radiation Physics and Protection, Oxford University Hospitals NHS FT, Oxford, UK

[5] Department of Biomedical Engineering, School of Biomedical Engineering and Imaging Sciences, King's College London, London, UK

Abstract. Tumor heterogeneity can be assessed quantitatively by analyzing dynamic contrast-enhanced imaging modalities potentially leading to improvement in the diagnosis and treatment of cancer, for example of the lung. However, the acquisition of standard lung sequences is often compromised by irregular breathing motion artefacts, resulting in unsystematic errors when estimating tissue perfusion parameters. In this work, we illustrate implicit deformable image registration that integrates the Demons algorithm using the local correlation coefficient as a similarity measure, and locally adaptive regularization that enables incorporation of both spatial sliding motions and irregular temporal motion patterns. We also propose a practical numerical approximation of the regularization model to improve both computational time and registration accuracy, which are important when analyzing long clinical sequences. Our quantitative analysis of 4D lung Computed Tomography and Computed Tomography Perfusion scans from clinical lung trial shows significant improvement over state-of-the-art pairwise registration approaches.

1 Introduction

Dynamic imaging modalities such as Computed Tomography Perfusion (CTP) or Dynamic Contrast Enhanced Magnetic Resonance Imaging (DCE-MRI) have attracted significant interest in quantitative oncological imaging since they have the great potential for the assessment of tumor heterogeneity, leading, in turn, to improvements in diagnosis and the formulation of personalized patient treatment plan [5,10]. These dynamic modalities have been widely used in clinical applications related to brain [7] or head and neck radiotherapy [4], but their

© Springer International Publishing AG, part of Springer Nature 2018
S. Klein et al. (Eds.): WBIR 2018, LNCS 10883, pp. 37–46, 2018.
https://doi.org/10.1007/978-3-319-92258-4_4

application has been rather limited in lung and abdominal radiotherapy, not least because of the deformations caused primarily by breathing [20]. The complexity of human lung motion and the irregular temporal motion patterns rule out generic deformable image registration methods as they are unable to model accurately the properties of the relevant tissues. Therefore, modeling and analyzing lung and abdominal motion has been recognized as an important element of many biomedical image analysis applications [16].

1.1   Related Work

The standard approach to motion correction of dynamic sequences is to perform state-of-the-art pairwise deformable registration algorithms [17] between the reference and the follow-up volumes from a sequence. While such an approach is straightforward, it results in inverse inconsistency and transitivity errors [6] of the estimated transformations due to accumulation of errors in the sequence. Such errors are then propagated to any subsequent pharmacokinetic analysis. Additionally, there is bias introduced in the registration results due to the selection of a fixed reference volume, since choosing an outlying reference volume may be disadvantageous as all registrations will need to estimate inadequate large displacement fields. To reduce errors related to estimation of the displacement fields, numerous methods have incorporated temporal smoothness constraints [1,2,12,18]. However, temporal regularization models do not solve the problem of the fixed reference volume, and so temporal groupwise image registration has been proposed [13,21,22]. Simultaneous registration of all images in a sequence reduces the bias introduced by a fixed reference volume, while temporal regularization preserves smoothness of the estimated displacement fields. Although such an approach is more robust to outliers, temporal smoothness is implausible for irregular motion artefacts, which are apparent for patients with lung cancer or other co-morbidities.

Contributions. We explore groupwise deformable image registration [22] to dynamic lung Computed Tomography (CT) as a method that is intrinsically invariant to the selection of reference volume and irregularity of lung expiration/inspiration motion pattern. In particular, we developed a groupwise deformable image registration derived from the LCC Demons [11] with adaptive regularization using local spatial and temporal filtering of the estimated displacement fields [14]. The main contributions of the manuscript are as follows: we extend 3D guided image filtering to its 4D counterpart to enable efficient spatio-temporal regularization of the estimated displacement fields from groupwise image registration. Guided image filtering [9] is a computationally attractive, linear image filtering technique, and here we used it to propagate spatio-temporal information from a so-called guidance image to the regularization. We present a numerical approximation which significantly reduces the computational burden whilst improving registration accuracy, which is important when dealing with large 4D data set. The improved performance on a publicly available lung

CT data set [3] is quantitatively assessed. Finally, the robustness of the method on a challenging clinical application of CTP motion compensation for patients with non-small cell lung cancer is demonstrated.

2   Methods

2.1   Classic Groupwise Deformable Image Registration

In the classic formulation [6], groupwise deformable image registration is defined as a global energy minimization problem:

$$\hat{\mathbf{u}} = \arg\min_{\boldsymbol{u}} \left(\varepsilon(\boldsymbol{u}) = Sim(\mathbf{I}(\boldsymbol{u})) + \alpha Reg(\boldsymbol{u})\right) \tag{1}$$

with respect to a set of displacement fields $\boldsymbol{u}$ describing geometrical correspondences between a set of M input images $\mathbf{I} = [I_m : \Omega \rightarrow \mathbb{R}, \Omega \in \mathbb{R}^3, m = 1, \ldots M]$. If a reference image I_{ref} for groupwise deformable image registration is explicitly provided, the process of estimation of the set of displacement fields to such a reference image is called reference-based groupwise registration and the objective function ε is defined as follows:

$$\varepsilon(\boldsymbol{u}) = \sum_{m=1}^{M} Sim(I_{ref}, I_m(\boldsymbol{u}_m)) + \alpha \sum_{m=1}^{M} Reg(\boldsymbol{u}_m) \tag{2}$$

In the case when the reference image I_{ref} is not provided, the estimation of the set of the displacement fields from each image I_m in the set $\mathbf{I}$ is performed with respect to the unknown reference image, considering minimization the sum of the similarity measure Sim between each pair of the input images as follows:

$$\varepsilon(\boldsymbol{u}) = \sum_{m=1}^{M} \sum_{\substack{n=1 \\ n \neq m}}^{M} Sim(I_m(\boldsymbol{u}_m), I_n(\boldsymbol{u}_n)) + \alpha \sum_{m=1}^{M} Reg(\boldsymbol{u}_m) \tag{3}$$

The objective function of the implicit groupwise deformable image registration defined by Eq. (3) can be solved using a variety of methods. Because of its simplicity and efficiency, we choose the Demons framework [19] to solve Eq. (3). For the Demons framework, the optimization procedure alternates between minimizing the energy related to the similarity measure Sim and the regularization Reg in an iterative manner. The contributions of this work will be described in detail in the following sections.

2.2   Groupwise Similarity Measure

From the fact that the symmetric image registration can be seen as an implicit groupwise image registration with only two input images, the minimization process of groupwise registration (Eq. (3)) is similar to the symmetric registration [11]. In the standard Demons registration, the displacement field is estimated by the minimization of the sum of the squared differences (SSD) between the input images. In the case of the time scans acquired with contrast agent, the SSD is not viable choice since it is not robust to the local intensity changes caused by wash-in and wash-out of contrast. Here, we propose to replace SSD-based groupwise registration to the local correlation coefficient (LCC) based counterpart. LCC-Demons has already been used for symmetric brain MRI registration due to the independence of any additive and multiplicative noise in the data [11]. The LCC similarity measure between a pair of images I_1 and I_2 defined for symmetric registration is defined in the following way:

$$LCC(I_1(u_1), I_2(u_2)) = \frac{\bar{I}_1(u_1)\bar{I}_2(u_2)}{(\bar{I}_1(u_1))^2(\bar{I}_2(u_2))^2} \quad (4)$$

where $\bar{I}_1$ and $\bar{I}_2$ are the local mean image intensities for image I_1 and I_2, respectively. Following the derivation in [11], the LCC symmetric update of the displacement field for the Demons can be calculated with a closed form formula as follows:

$$du_{12}(x) = \frac{-2force_{lcc}}{(force_{lcc} + \sigma_{noise}^2)} \quad (5)$$

at any spatial position x in the image domain, σ_{noise}^2 is a noise estimator, and

$$force_{lcc} = G * \left(\frac{I_1 \nabla I_2^T}{I_1 I_2} - \frac{I_2 \nabla I_1^T}{I_1 I_2} + \frac{I_1 \nabla I_1^T}{I_1^2} - \frac{I_2 \nabla I_2^T}{I_2^2} \right) \quad (6)$$

where $G*$ is a Gaussian kernel for smoothing. Finally, the average update of the displacement field for the groupwise registration is calculated using the log-Euclidean mean for vector field $du(x)$ given by:

$$du_m(x) = \frac{1}{M-1} \sum_{\substack{n=1 \\ n \neq m}}^{M} (du_{mn}(x)) \quad (7)$$

2.3 Spatio-Temporal Filtering of Displacement Fields

Motion correction for intra-subject dynamic imaging of lungs is challenging due to the complexity of motion to be estimated stemming from patient breathing during acquisition. The standard regularization model of the Demons framework realized by Gaussian smoothing of the estimated displacement field has been shown to be inadequate to model respiratory motion. Here, we extend a previous approach [14], where spatially adaptive filtering of displacement field using the guided image filtering technique was developed, and we present a generic approach for 4D regularization. In our approach, the estimated displacement field is additionally filtered by considering the temporal context of the guidance information encoded in the dynamic imaging.

Following [14, 15], the initial displacement field u_{in} is first spatially filtered considering the context of the guidance information I_g as follows:

$$u_{tmp}(x) = \sum_{y \in \mathcal{N}} W_{spatial}(I_g, x, y)(u_{in}(y) + du_m(y)) \quad (8)$$

where $\mathcal{N}$ is the local spatial neighborhood (a box window of size $r_\mathcal{N}$), and $W_{spatial}$ are the kernel weights for spatial filter. Similarly, the filtered displacement field $\boldsymbol{u}_{tmp}$ is then temporally filtered again using the dynamic context of the guidance information $I_g(t)$ in the following way:

$$\boldsymbol{u}_{out}(\boldsymbol{x}) = \sum_{t\in\mathcal{T}} W_{temporal}\left(I_g, \boldsymbol{x}, t\right)\left(\boldsymbol{u}_{tmp}(\boldsymbol{x}, t) + \boldsymbol{du}_m(\boldsymbol{x}, t)\right) \tag{9}$$

where $\mathcal{T}$ is the local temporal neighborhood (a box window of size $r_\mathcal{T}$), and $W_{temporal}$ are the kernel weights for temporal filter.

Our regularization method is composed of two main steps: spatial adaptive filtering of the displacement field to enforce discontinuity preserving properties at lung interfaces; and adaptive temporal filtering of the displacement field to ensure capture of temporal (ir)regularities of the patient's motion pattern. In our framework, these two steps could not be combined in one step of filtering the estimated displacement field, because the local spatial neighborhood and the local temporal neighborhood have different units, and respective parameters $r_\mathcal{N}$ and $r_\mathcal{T}$ need to be setup separately.

Regularization with Subsampled Guided Image Filter. Since medical volumes can easily be $512 \times 512 \times 120$ or larger, a linear time (with respect of the number of voxels) can be still considered to be computationally significant, particularly since the filtering procedure is repeated at every iteration of the presented deformable registration. Therefore, we adapt a speed-up strategy for fast guided filters mentioned in [8] to improve performance of the presented filtering-based regularization. Most of the computation time for the guided filters is spent on the estimation of the filter coefficients, however the coefficients do not need to be estimated from full-resolution volumes. Therefore, to estimate those coefficients, we subsample the input and guidance image by factor s, and perform all computations related to filtering of the displacement on the subsampled volumes. Then, the coefficients estimated from the subsampled volumes are upsampled to the original size of the volumes, and then the final step of guided filtering is performed using the original guidance image I_G and the upsampled coefficients. Due to the use of a subsampled image to estimate the filter coefficients, the computational cost of filtering can be reduced approximately by s^2 as only the final step is performed on full size volume. Comparison of the influence of filtering of the estimated displacement using the subsampled volumes is shown in Sect. 3.2.

3 Experiments

3.1 Data Description

For quantitative evaluation of the proposed regularization method we use a publicly available 4D CT data set [3]. The *Dir-Lab* data set consists of 10 consecutive respiratory cycle phase volumes with spatial resolution varying between

$0.97 \times 0.97 \times 2.5$ and $1.16 \times 1.16 \times 2.5 \, mm^3$. To quantify registration accuracy, the Target Registration Error (TRE) was calculated for the well-distributed set of landmarks, which are provided with this data set (300 landmarks per case for inhale and exhale volumes).

For the second experiment, the method was evaluated on CTP data from a clinical trial (NCT02628080) acquired at the Churchill Hospital in Oxford evaluating whether an investigational drug (atovaquone) alters tumour hypoxia. The data reported here are for the pre-atovaquone scans. For the CTP patients are imaged supine on a GE Discovery 710 PET/CT scanner with a 45s cine mode CT using 120 kV and 60 mA. During this 70 mL contrast (Omnipaque 300) is injected at 5 mL/s followed by 25 mL water at 5 mL/s. The patient is instructed to hold their breath for as long as possible (at inspiration) and if necessary to breathe out very slowly.

3.2   Results for Publicly Available 4D Lung CT Dataset

Table 1 shows the TRE based on 300 well-populated, manually annotated landmarks for all ten cases included in the Dir-Lab data set [3]. The initial TRE is $8.46 \pm 5.5 \, mm$ and the transformations estimated by the proposed method with subsampling factor $s = 4$ reduces the TRE to $1.47 \pm 0.5 \, mm$, achieving the best result in our comparison.

Table 1. Results achieved by the proposed method with different value of the subsampling factor s for 4D registration of CT lung from Dir-Lab data set. The method with the subsampling factor $s = 4$ shows the lowest average Target Registration Error (TRE) among all methods.

	Before	Subsampling factor s					
		$s = 1$ [14]	$s = 2$	$s = 3$	$s = 4$	$s = 5$	$s = 6$
$c1$	3.89 ± 2.9	0.95 ± 0.9	1.08 ± 1.1	0.88 ± 1.0	0.90 ± 1.0	$\mathbf{0.86 \pm 1.0}$	$\mathbf{0.86 \pm 1.0}$
$c2$	4.34 ± 3.9	0.95 ± 1.0	1.00 ± 1.0	0.98 ± 1.1	0.94 ± 1.0	$\mathbf{0.91 \pm 1.0}$	0.92 ± 1.0
$c3$	6.94 ± 4.1	1.06 ± 1.1	1.09 ± 1.1	$\mathbf{1.03 \pm 1.1}$	1.06 ± 1.1	1.08 ± 1.1	1.27 ± 1.2
$c4$	9.83 ± 4.9	3.19 ± 4.8	3.16 ± 4.3	2.71 ± 3.7	$\mathbf{2.53 \pm 3.2}$	2.62 ± 3.1	2.70 ± 3.0
$c5$	7.48 ± 5.5	1.40 ± 1.5	1.44 ± 1.6	1.33 ± 1.5	$\mathbf{1.31 \pm 1.5}$	1.41 ± 1.5	1.51 ± 1.5
$c6$	10.9 ± 7.0	2.74 ± 3.2	2.63 ± 3.2	2.19 ± 2.5	1.89 ± 1.9	$\mathbf{1.82 \pm 1.6}$	1.88 ± 1.4
$c7$	11.0 ± 7.4	1.69 ± 1.6	1.67 ± 1.6	$\mathbf{1.52 \pm 1.4}$	$\mathbf{1.52 \pm 1.4}$	1.74 ± 1.6	1.91 ± 1.4
$c8$	15.0 ± 9.0	2.45 ± 3.1	2.10 ± 2.6	$\mathbf{1.85 \pm 2.3}$	1.87 ± 2.3	2.02 ± 2.4	2.35 ± 2.4
$c9$	7.92 ± 4.0	1.56 ± 1.0	$\mathbf{1.31 \pm 1.2}$	1.33 ± 1.1	1.37 ± 1.1	1.55 ± 1.2	1.79 ± 1.2
$c10$	7.30 ± 6.4	1.46 ± 1.8	1.40 ± 1.7	1.36 ± 1.5	$\mathbf{1.27 \pm 1.4}$	1.29 ± 1.3	1.43 ± 1.3
$T\tilde{R}E$	8.46 ± 5.5	1.71 ± 0.8	1.69 ± 0.7	1.52 ± 0.6	$\mathbf{1.47 \pm 0.5}$	1.53 ± 0.5	1.66 ± 0.6

Visualization of the results for the presented method is shown in Fig. 1. Red arrows depict regions of interest where the presented method with the subsampling factor $s = 4$ outperformed the baseline method with the subsampling factor $s = 1$.

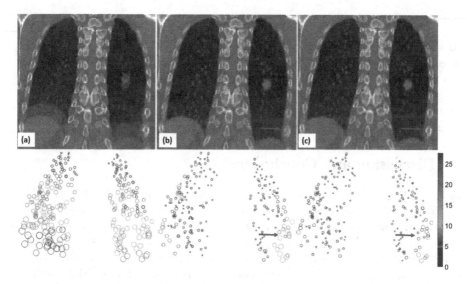

Fig. 1. Visualization of the image intensity differences (top) and 2D projection of the Target Registration Error (bottom) before registration (a), and after performing the proposed method with the subsampling factor (b) $s = 1$ [14], and (c) $s = 4$ for the challenging case 6 from Dir-Lab. Color overlay is given for the coronal view of inhale (green) and exhale (magenta) volumes. TRE is projected on the coronal plane and denoted by the size and color of circles. A clear improvement after registration using the presented method is visible (labeled by red arrows). (Color figure online)

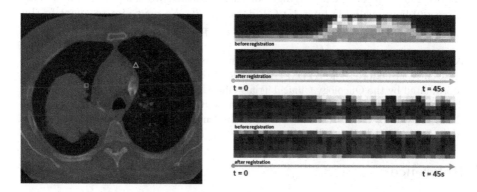

Fig. 2. Axial (left) view for reference volume with cyan and magenta pointers indicating the locations of their corresponding time-cuts for CTP in the challenging case $\#AT010$ before and after registration using the proposed method with the subsampling factor (b) $s = 4$.

3.3 Results for Lung Tumor CTP

At the time of writing, we have analyzed 11 dynamic 4D-CTP scans of patients who have a lung tumor. Registration quality was evaluated via the Correlation Coefficient (CC), and for all data sets, and noticeable improvement was found (avg. CC before = 0.96, and after = 0.99). Figure 2 shows an axial view of an exemplar CTP and the time-cuts, which demonstrate visual improvement in alignment over acquisition time of CTP volumes.

4   Discussion and Conclusions

In this paper, we have presented a new class of 4D regularization model based on 4D guided image filtering, that can be easily incorporated into groupwise deformable image registration. Furthermore, we have shown that the use of the subsampled guided image to calculate the filter's coefficient for the displacement fields improves the registration accuracy while reduces computational cost of registration. This is particularly important for long temporal acquisitions such as DCE-MRI or CTP, which consists of several volumes. From a clinical perspective, our registration framework compensates for misalignment between consecutive CTP volumes caused by patient-specific breath-hold variability, resulting in the improved alignment of structure of interest in the lungs. We obtained a good visual alignment of the CTP data, however actual registration errors measured by the densely distributed landmarks was not assessed. Manual annotations of temporal functional imaging e.g. Computed Tomography Perfusion is inevitably labor-intensive. Furthermore, intensity changes caused by contrast uptake or the low contrast of lung tissue in Computed Tomography Perfusion makes accurate annotation even more challenging. For these reasons, we compared our method using publicly available lung 4D CT data set [3]. We next aim to quantify the impact of our method on estimation of tissue perfusion parameters.

Acknowledgments. We acknowledge funding from the CRUK/EPSRC Cancer Imaging Centre in Oxford. The ATOM trial is sponsored by the University of Oxford and coordinated by the Oncology Clinical Trials Office. It is supported by the Howat Foundation, Oxford Cancer Imaging Centre, Cancer Research UK, National Institute of Health Research, Oxford Biomedical Research Centre and the ECMC. BWP acknowledges Oxford NIHR Biomedical Research Centre (Rutherford Fund).

References

1. Bai, W., Brady, M.: Regularized B-spline deformable registration for respiratory motion correction in PET images. Phys. Med. Biol. **54**(9), 2719 (2009)
2. Castillo, E., Castillo, R., Martinez, J., Shenoy, M., Guerrero, T.: Four-dimensional deformable image registration using trajectory modeling. Phys. Med. Biol. **55**(1), 305 (2009)
3. Castillo, R., Castillo, E., Guerra, R., Johnson, V., McPhail, T., Garg, A., Guerrero, T.: A framework for evaluation of deformable image registration spatial accuracy using large landmark point sets. Phys. Med. Biol. **54**, 1849–1870 (2009)

4. Craciunescu, O.I., Yoo, D.S., Cleland, E., Muradyan, N., Carroll, M.D., MacFall, J.R., Barboriak, D.P., Brizel, D.M.: Dynamic contrast-enhanced MRI in head-and-neck cancer: the impact of region of interest selection on the intra-and interpatient variability of pharmacokinetic parameters. Int. J. Radiat. Oncol. Biol. Phys. **82**(3), e345–e350 (2012)
5. García-Figueiras, R., Goh, V.J., Padhani, A.R., Baleato-González, S., Garrido, M., León, L., Gómez-Caamaño, A.: CT perfusion in oncologic imaging: a useful tool? Am. J. Roentgenol. **200**(1), 8–19 (2013)
6. Geng, X., Christensen, G.E., Gu, H., Ross, T.J., Yang, Y.: Implicit reference-based group-wise image registration and its application to structural and functional MRI. Neuroimage **47**(4), 1341–1351 (2009)
7. Godenschweger, F., Kägebein, U., Stucht, D., Yarach, U., Sciarra, A., Yakupov, R., Lüsebrink, F., Schulze, P., Speck, O.: Motion correction in MRI of the brain. Phys. Med. Biol. **61**(5), R32 (2016)
8. He, K., Sun, J.: Fast guided filter. arXiv preprint arXiv:1505.00996 (2015)
9. He, K., Sun, J., Tang, X.: Guided image filtering. IEEE Trans. Pattern Anal. Mach. Intell. **35**(6), 1397–1409 (2013)
10. Koyama, H., Ohno, Y., Seki, S., Nishio, M., Yoshikawa, T., Matsumoto, S., Sugimura, K.: Magnetic resonance imaging for lung cancer. J. Thorac. Imaging **28**(3), 138–150 (2013)
11. Lorenzi, M., Ayache, N., Frisoni, G.B., Pennec, X., Alzheimer's Disease Neuroimaging Initiative (ADNI): LCC-Demons: a robust and accurate symmetric diffeomorphic registration algorithm. Neuroimage **81**, 470–483 (2013)
12. McClelland, J.R., Blackall, J.M., Tarte, S., Chandler, A.C., Hughes, S., Ahmad, S., Landau, D.B., Hawkes, D.J.: A continuous 4D motion model from multiple respiratory cycles for use in lung radiotherapy. Med. Phys. **33**(9), 3348–3358 (2006)
13. Metz, C.T., Klein, S., Schaap, M., van Walsum, T., Niessen, W.J.: Nonrigid registration of dynamic medical imaging data using nD+ t B-splines and a groupwise optimization approach. Med. Image Anal. **15**(2), 238–249 (2011)
14. Papież, B.W., Franklin, J., Heinrich, M.P., Gleeson, F.V., Schnabel, J.A.: Liver motion estimation via locally adaptive over-segmentation regularization. In: Navab, N., Hornegger, J., Wells, W.M., Frangi, A.F. (eds.) MICCAI 2015. LNCS, vol. 9351, pp. 427–434. Springer, Cham (2015). https://doi.org/10.1007/978-3-319-24574-4_51
15. Papież, B.W., Heinrich, M.P., Fehrenbach, J., Risser, L., Schnabel, J.A.: An implicit sliding-motion preserving regularisation via bilateral filtering for deformable image registration. Med. Image Anal. **18**(8), 1299–1311 (2014)
16. Schnabel, J.A., Heinrich, M.P., Papież, B.W., Brady, J.M.: Advances and challenges in deformable image registration: from image fusion to complex motion modelling. Med. Image Anal. **33**, 145–148 (2016)
17. Sotiras, A., Davatzikos, C., Paragios, N.: Deformable medical image registration: a survey. IEEE Trans. Med. Imaging **32**(7), 1153–1190 (2013)
18. Vandemeulebroucke, J., Rit, S., Kybic, J., Clarysse, P., Sarrut, D.: Spatiotemporal motion estimation for respiratory-correlated imaging of the lungs. Med. Phys. **38**(1), 166–178 (2011)
19. Vercauteren, T., Pennec, X., Perchant, A., Ayache, N.: Diffeomorphic demons: efficient non-parametric image registration. Neuroimage **45**, S61–S72 (2009)
20. von Siebenthal, M., Szekely, G., Gamper, U., Boesiger, P., Lomax, A., Cattin, P.: 4D MR imaging of respiratory organ motion and its variability. Phys. Med. Biol. **52**(6), 1547 (2007)

21. Wu, G., Wang, Q., Shen, D., Alzheimer's Disease NeuroImaging Initiative, et al.: Registration of longitudinal brain image sequences with implicit template and spatial-temporal heuristics. NeuroImage **59**(1), 404–421 (2012)
22. Yigitsoy, M., Wachinger, C., Navab, N.: Temporal groupwise registration for motion modeling. In: Székely, G., Hahn, H.K. (eds.) IPMI 2011. LNCS, vol. 6801, pp. 648–659. Springer, Heidelberg (2011). https://doi.org/10.1007/978-3-642-22092-0_53

A Novel Similarity Measure for Image Sequences

Kai Brehmer[1]([✉]), Benjamin Wacker[1], and Jan Modersitzki[1,2]

[1] Institute of Mathematics and Image Computing, University of Lübeck,
Lübeck, Germany
brehmer@mic.uni-luebeck.de
[2] Fraunhofer MEVIS, Lübeck, Germany

Abstract. Quantification of image similarity is a common problem in image processing. For pairs of two images, a variety of options is available and well-understood. However, some applications such as dynamic imaging or serial sectioning involve the analysis of image sequences and thus require a simultaneous and unbiased comparison of many images.

This paper proposes a new similarity measure, that takes a global perspective and involves all images at the same time. The key idea is to look at Schatten-q-norms of a matrix assembled from normalized gradient fields of the image sequence. In particular, for $q = 0$, the measure is minimized if the gradient information from the image sequence has a low rank.

This global perspective of the novel SqN-measure does not only allow to register sequences from dynamic imaging, e.g. DCE-MRI, but is also a new opportunity to simultaneously register serial sections, e.g. in histology. In this way, an accumulation of small, local registration errors may be avoided.

First numerical experiments show very promising results for a DCE-MRI sequence of a human kidney as well as for a set of serial sections. The global structure of the data used for registration with SqN is preserved in all cases.

1 Introduction

Quantification of image similarity is a common problem in image processing. For pairs of two images, a variety of options such as sum of squared differences (SSD), normalized gradient fields (NGF), or mutual information (MI) exists and these measures are well-understood; see e.g. [12,13,17]. However, some applications such as dynamic imaging or serial sectioning involve the analysis of image sequences and thus require a simultaneous and unbiased comparison of many images.

In some of these applications, image intensity may changes over time. For example, the glomerular filtration rate (GFR) is an important parameter for kidney malfunction [18]. The GFR might be determined on the basis of a time series of dynamic contrast-enhanced magnetic resonance images (DCE-MRI).

© Springer International Publishing AG, part of Springer Nature 2018
S. Klein et al. (Eds.): WBIR 2018, LNCS 10883, pp. 47–56, 2018.
https://doi.org/10.1007/978-3-319-92258-4_5

This sequence then needs to be registered in order to correct for motion artifacts; see, e.g., [7,9]. Another example is the analysis of a histological serial sectioning. Here, the staining of sections might be different and/or can express severe variations.

For applications like these, a proper image similarity measure is crucial. A standard approach is to perform a sequential comparison of pairs of two images from the sequence. However, a sequential registration is restricted to local rather than global information. Moreover, there might be issues choosing a suited starting image and determining the order of the sequence. Results may depend on these choices. There also exists a variety of statistical approaches for global image registration; see e.g. [5,10,16,21]. However, we focus on a new global measure which is based on deterministic image features.

In this paper, we propose the new SqN similarity measure, that is designed to compare a complete image sequence simultaneously and thus automatically distributing information in a global way. Our key idea is to look at Schatten-q-norms (more precisely: Schatten-q-quasinorms) of a matrix that is assembled from normalized gradient fields of the image sequence. Particularly for $q = 0$, the measure is minimized for sequences of images where the gradient matrix has low rank and the approach is thus connected to principal component analysis and sparsity.

Our idea is motivated from color image denoising; see Möllenhoff et al. [14]. In that context, similar concepts are used as a regularization for TV denoising, and the gradient matrix is formed directly from gradients of the three color channels. In our paper, we interpret the individual images from a sequence as individual channels and use a Schatten-q-norm of the matrix of normalized gradients as a data fitting term rather than as a regularizer. As we will show, this can be viewed as a natural extension of NGF [6] and can thus deal with multi-modal frames. We remark that the concept also relates to ideas in video compression.

Our paper is organized as follows: At first we describe the novel distance measure and its relation to NGF as well as its characteristics. Moreover, we show numerical results for DCE-MRI time series and a H&E stained histological serial section of a mouse brain. We compare the performance of SqN with NGF (DCE-MRI) and the well-known SSD (serial sectioning). Our examples show that SqN results at least comparable registration results but is about six times faster as the competitive approaches. To conclude our paper, we discuss the numerical results and give a brief outlook on what our next steps are.

2   The Novel Similarity Measure SqN

Our new distance measure is motivated by a regularizer for color image denoising; see [14]. The underlying idea is that in natural images, gradients of the different color channels are linearly dependent; see also Fig. 1. Therefore, an appropriate measure of dependency such as Schatten-q-norms [24] are excellent regularizers in color image denoising. This idea can be generalized to more than three channels and is therefore useful in applications such as parameter estimation in DCE-MRI [8] or the registration of multiple images as they appear for example in serial sectioning or time series [11].

We motivate our extension starting with a conceptual simpler but computational infeasible approach. The main point is to motivate the use of Schatten-q-norms. We then present a computational tractable version that is based on local image gradients. In contrast to [14] where a similar measure is used as regularizer, we also propose to use our new functional as a distance measure.

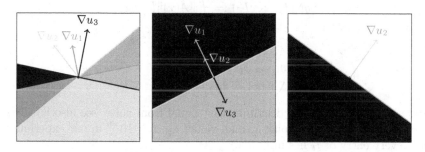

Fig. 1. Illustration of a local gradient matrix $A = [\nabla u_1, \nabla u_2, \nabla u_3] \in \mathbb{R}^{2,3}$ of three color channels; illustration adapted from [14]. The rank of A is two (left) or one (center and right).

We recall that any matrix $A \in \mathbb{R}^{n,T}$ has a singular value decomposition (SVD) [4],

$$A = U\mathrm{diag}(S)V^\top, \text{ with } U^\top U = E_n,\ V^\top V = E_T.$$

Here, E_d denotes the d-by-d identity matrix, $S = (\sigma_1, \ldots, \sigma_{\min\{n,T\}})$ is a vector with ordered entries $\sigma_j \geq \sigma_{j+1} \geq 0$ and $\mathrm{diag}(S) \in \mathbb{R}^{n,T}$ denotes a diagonal matrix. Using the SVD, the Schatten-q-(quasi)-norm of A is then defined as

$$\|A\|_{S,q}^q := \|S\|_q^q = \sum_i \sigma_i^q \quad \text{for} \quad q \geq 0.$$

An optimal choice of q is obviously application dependent. In particular for registration problems, it is topic of current research. Note that for $q = 0$, the measure counts non-zero entries and is not a norm but a so-called quasinorm. With $q = 0$, we thus promote sparsity of S and hence low rank of A. However, optimization of the 0-quasinorm is non-trivial and it is typically replaced by the minimization of the 1-norm; see [2]. Following [14], we use $q = 1/2$ in this paper.

We are now ready to describe our novel similarity measure. To this end, we assume that $T \in \mathbb{N}$ discrete images I_t are given, where each I_t is of dimension $m_1 \times \cdots \times m_d \in \mathbb{N}^d$ and $d \in \mathbb{N}$ denotes the spatial dimension. Let $n := m_1 \cdots m_d$ and I_t be reshaped as $n \times 1$ array. The first idea is to look at the rank of $A = [I_1, \ldots, I_T] \in \mathbb{R}^{n,T}$ as an indicator for the linear dependency of the images.

Note that this approach is similar to a principal component analysis of the data. However, this approach is not suitable for images with varying intensities such as DCE-MRI or serial sections. Although this approach is conceptually appealing, it is computationally challenging as the complexity of the SVD is $\mathcal{O}\left(\min\{nT^2, Tn^2\}\right)$ [4].

We escape the complexity problem by applying the measure to local structures. More precisely, we define our new distance measure SqN for a sequence of T images by

$$\mathrm{SqN}(I_1, \ldots, I_T) := \int \|A(x)\|_{S,q}^q \, dx,$$

where

$$A(x) := [\eta_1, \ldots, \eta_T] \in \mathbb{R}^{d,T} \quad \text{and}$$
$$\eta_t := (\nabla I_t(x)^\top \nabla I_t(x) + \eta^2)^{-1/2} \, \nabla I_t(x).$$

Here, $\eta > 0$ is a parameter discriminating signal from noise; see also [6]. If the noise level is unknown, we pick a small value, e.g. $\eta = 10^{-5}$ in our experiments where every entry of I_t lies in $[0, 256)$.

We now outline the connection to NGF [6]. For two images I_1 and I_2, fixed x, $\eta = 0$ and with $\alpha := |\cos\angle(\nabla I_1, \nabla I_2)|$, we have

$$A^\top A = \begin{pmatrix} 1 & \alpha \\ \alpha & 1 \end{pmatrix} \text{ with singular values } \sigma_1^2 = 1 + \alpha \text{ and } \sigma_2^2 = 1 - \alpha.$$

Particularly for $q = 0$, the distance is minimal if the image gradients are collinear, i.e. $\alpha = 1$. Therefore, our new measure might be interpreted as a generalization of the normalized gradient field based distance measure [6]. Analogous arguments hold for $0 \leq q < 2$. Remarkably, for $q = 2$, the energy function is constant and the measure thus meaningless. For $q > 2$, the function is minimal for perpendicular gradients.

3   Numerical Results for Dynamic Imaging and Serial Sections

We now present results for the registration of DCE-MRI sequences of a human kidney and a histological serial sectioning of a mouse brain.

We start with registrations of DCE-MRI sequences of a human kidney; data courtesy of Jarle Rørvik, Haukeland University Hospital Bergen, Norway. Here, 3D images are taken at 49 time points. The objective is to register the images while maintaining the dynamics. More precisely, we use 146-by-82 coronal slices of a 146-by-82-by-52-by-49 volume for z-Slice 25; see Fig. 2.

Our registration scheme is based on the variational image registration framework FAIR [13]. More precisely, we minimize

$$\mathcal{J}(y_1, \ldots, y_T) = \mathrm{SqN}(I_1(y_1), \ldots, I_T(y_T)) + \alpha \sum_{t=1}^{T} \mathcal{S}(y_t).$$

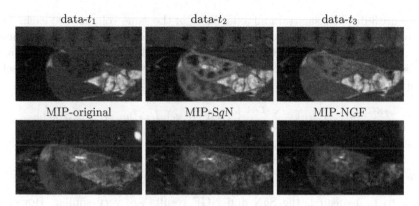

Fig. 2. DCE-MRI data of a human kidney; data courtesy of Jarle Rørvik, Haukeland University Hospital Bergen, Norway. Top row: Displayed are 2D slices at three representative time points during contrast agent uptake. Images are rotated by 90 degrees for presentation purposes. Bottom row: Coronal view of maximum intensity projections $\sum_{j>i} |I_j - I_i|$ for original, SqN-registered, and NGF-registered data. Note the blurred and doubled structures in the non-registered data.

For ease of presentation, we use the curvature regularizer $\mathcal{S}(y) = \int (\Delta y)^2 \, dx$ with regularization parameter $\alpha = 0.1$ [1]. Optimization is performed in a standard way using a Gauß-Newton algorithm with Armijo linesearch [15] within a multilevel framework [13]. All computations are performed using MATLAB.

Figure 2 (top row) shows three representative coronal slices of the original dataset. The slices correspond to different times during acquisition. Different phases of contrast agent uptake are visible, particularly within the kidney.

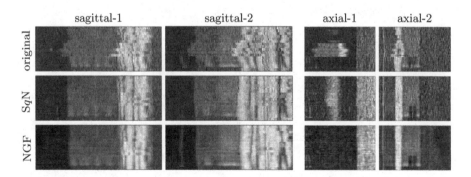

Fig. 3. Two exemplary sagittal and axial slices of the data, each; see also Fig. 2. Original, non-registered data (top row), SqN-registered data (middle row, $q = 0.5$), and NGF-registered data (bottom row), $\eta = 25$. Note that the laminar structure of the tissue is only visible after registration. The axial sections in this visualization do not necessarily correspond.

Figure 3 displays sagittal and axial slices of the same volume, two each. The top row shows non-registered slices where motion artefacts are clearly visible. The middle row shows corresponding SqN-registration results for $q = 0.5$ and the bottom row shows results for sequential NGF, respectively. More precisely, we optimized

$$\mathcal{J}^{\text{NGF}}(y_1, \ldots, y_T) = \sum_{t=1}^{T-1} \left\{ \text{NGF}(I_t(y_t), I_{t+1}(y_{t+1})) + \alpha\, \mathcal{S}(y_t) \right\}$$

using alternating optimization, i.e.

$$y_t^{k+1} = \text{argmin}_{y_t}\, \mathcal{J}^{\text{NGF}}(y_1^{k+1}, \ldots, y_{t-1}^{k+1},\, y_t,\, y_{t+1}^k, \ldots, y_T^k), \quad t = 1, \ldots, T.$$

As to be expected, the SqN and NGF results are very similar. However, within our non-optimized MATLAB framework, the SqN-registration is about

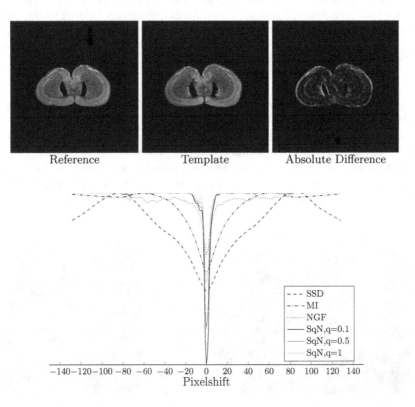

Reference   Template   Absolute Difference

Fig. 4. Results for a translation of two stained histological serial sections; data courtesy of O. Schmitt, University of Rostock, Germany [19]. The top row displays the similar slices 160 (reference) and 170 (template) of a stack of 189 slices in total as well as the absolute difference image. The bottom row displays the corresponding energies of the different distance measures listed in the legend. The images used for translation are of size 256×256 pixel. The y axis of the graphs are scaled individually for better comparison.

six times faster than the NGF registration — even if the alternating optimization approach is limited to a forward-backward sweep.

Figure 2 also illustrates the intensity variations in the original and registered data. It is apparent that intensity variations due to motion have been reduced tremendously. Note that the variations, in particular in kidney and bladder (partly visible), are still visible and therefore the schemes allow for a subsequent dynamical analysis.

The SqN measure is also capable of serial section registration. Figure 5 displays results for a H&E stained histological serial section of a mouse brain; 189 sections of 512-by-512 pixel; data courtesy of O. Schmitt, University of Rostock,

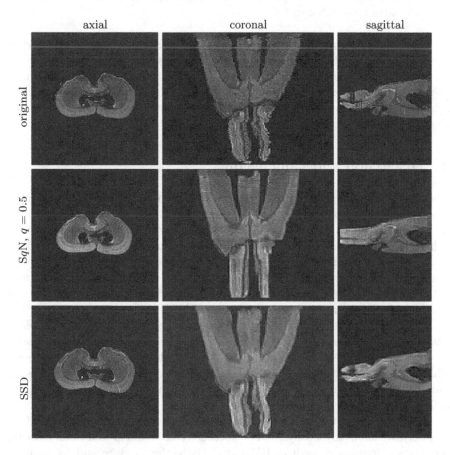

Fig. 5. Registration results for a stained histological serial sectioning; data courtesy of O. Schmitt, University of Rostock, Germany [19]. Displayed from left to right are exemplarily an axial, coronal, and sagittal slice of the 3D data of size 512-by-512-by-189. Displayed are non-registered data (top row), SqN-registered data (middle row) and SSD-registered data (bottom row). Note that the different slices do not necessarily correspond.

Germany; see [19] for experimental details. As this data has been normalized, we compare an SqN registration with a sequential SSD based approach. The figure displays the original data (top row), SqN results (middle row), and SSD results (bottom row). It is apparent that registration can reconstruct the local brain structure. Here, the SSD results appear to be slightly more blurred.

Note that a sequential approach involves an alternating optimization framework and is based on a fixed initial and final slice to avoid the so-called banana-effect [3,19,20,23], i.e. a global drift of structures due to sequential registration. The sequential registration process may accumulate small errors that can cause a major drift of the overall structure; see [23] for examples.

In contrast, the SqN approach enables a global optimization which in addition can be performed in just one pass. Moreover, our experiments indicate that SqN does not introduce global drifts.

Figure 4 shows the results of a translation experiment for the distance measures SSD, MI, NGF as wells as for SqN for three different configurations of the parameter q. It is apparent that q has an impact on the global minimum of the energy in this experiment. All measures have the same minimizer which is achieved for the template image in its origin when it is not shifted as shown in the difference image of Fig. 4.

4   Discussion and Conclusions

The novel SqN image similarity measure has been proposed. The new measure is motivated from color image denoising [14]. The main idea is to quantify structural image information expressed by normalized intensity gradients with Schatten-q-(quasi)-norms. For $q = 0$, the measure quantifies sparsity, i.e. redundancy of information in an image sequence. Moreover, using the normalized gradient fields as structural information, the focus is on image structures and not on intensity. Therefore, the new measure is effective in a multi-modal setup and it might be interpreted as an extension of NGF [6].

The novel measure considers the image sequence as a whole and therefore has no bias towards a particular ordering, which is common in a sequential setup. Therefore, the new measure provides also a global information transport, which might be beneficial for particular applications. In particular, it omits an unwanted drift of structure as it is very common in sequential approaches; so-called banana-effect [20].

We show the potential of the new measure in a registration setup. More precisely, we show how easily the new measure can be integrated in an existing registration framework such as FAIR [13]. Both, the measure and its analytic derivative are computed and thus, efficient optimization techniques can be used.

Exemplarily, we demonstrate the power of the measure in a registration problem for a dynamic contrast enhanced MRI sequence and histological serial sectioning. As it turns out, the new scheme produces results of at least comparable quality much faster (about six times faster in our experiments).

Particularly for serial section registrations, we escape an additional iterative process on the sequences of sections and make use of global information transport.

Our next steps include to come up with a more efficient implementation which is suitable in a 3D setup. We remark that the main computational cost is not the computation of the SVD of the gradient matrix. This involves the computation of eigenvalues of a T-by-T matrix, where T is the number of images in the sequence. In particular, T does not dependent on the spatial dimension of the data or the spatial resolution. However, the computation of the gradient matrix A does.

Moreover, we will investigate the impact of the distance measure in the analysis of the dynamic information within the DCE-MRI setting. With this knowledge, we would be able to quantify an optimal choice for the parameter q. In our current experiments, it appears that the impact of q is rather small unless we pick values close to $q = 2$. We also will compare the measure to global statistical measures (e.g. [5,10,16,21]) already used in this field of registration and image processing.

An implementation of SqN will soon be available within the FAIR-Toolbox; see https://github.com/C4IR.

Acknowledgement.

SPONSORED BY THE

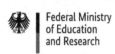

Federal Ministry
of Education
and Research

The authors acknowledge the financial support by the Federal Ministry of Education and Research of Germany in the framework of MED4D (project number 05M16FLA).

References

1. Fischer, B., Modersitzki, J.: Curvature based image registration. J. Math. Imaging Vis. **18**(1), 81–85 (2003)
2. Candes, E.J., Wakin, M.B., Boyd, S.: Enhancing sparsity by reweighted l_1 minimization. J. Fourier Anal. Appl. **14**(5), 877–905 (2008)
3. Gaffling, S., Daum, V., Hornegger, J.: Landmark-constrained 3-D histological imaging: a morphology-preserving approach. In: VMV, pp. 309–316 (2011)
4. Golub, G.H., Van Loan, C.F.: Matrix Computations, vol. 3. JHU Press, Baltimore (2012)
5. Guyader, J.M., et al.: Total correlation-based groupwise image registration for quantitative MRI. In: Proceedings of the IEEE Conference on Computer Vision and Pattern Recognition Workshops, pp. 186–193 (2016)
6. Haber, E., Modersitzki, J.: Beyond Mutual Information: a simple and robust alternative. In: Meinzer, H.P., Handels, H., Horsch, A., Tolxdorff, T. (eds.) Bildverarbeitung für die Medizin 2005. Informatik aktuell, pp. 350–354. Springer, Heidelberg (2005). https://doi.org/10.1007/3-540-26431-0_72

7. Heck, C., Ruthotto, L., Modersitzki, J., Berkels, B.: Model-based parameterestimation in DCE-MRI without an Arterial input function. In: Deserno, T.M., Handels, H., Meinzer, H.-P., Tolxdorff, T. (eds.) Bildverarbeitung für die Medizin 2014. I, pp. 246–251. Springer, Heidelberg (2014). https://doi.org/10.1007/978-3-642-54111-7_47

8. Heck, C., Benning, M., Modersitzki, J.: Joint registration and parameter estimation of T1 relaxation times using variable flip angles. In: Handels, H., Deserno, T.M., Meinzer, H.-P., Tolxdorff, T. (eds.) Bildverarbeitung für die Medizin 2015. I, pp. 215–220. Springer, Heidelberg (2015). https://doi.org/10.1007/978-3-662-46224-9_38

9. Hodneland, E., et al.: Segmentation-driven image registration-application to 4D DCE-MRI recordings of the moving kidneys. IEEE Trans. Image Process. **23**(5), 2392–2404 (2014)

10. Huizinga, W., et al.: PCA-based groupwise image registration for quantitative MRI. Med. Image Anal. **29**, 65–78 (2016)

11. Lotz, J., Berger, J., Müller, B., Breuhahn, K., et al.: Zooming in: high resolution 3D reconstruction of differently stained histological whole slide images, medical imaging 2014: digital pathology 9041: 904104. International Society for Optics and Photonics (2014)

12. Modersitzki, J.: Numerical Methods for Image Registration. Oxford University Press, Oxford (2004)

13. Modersitzki, J.: FAIR: flexible algorithms for image registration. Society for Industrial and Applied Mathematics (2009)

14. Möllenhoff, T., Strekalovskiy, E., Moeller, M., Cremers, D.: Low rank priors for color image regularization. In: Tai, X.-C., Bae, E., Chan, T.F., Lysaker, M. (eds.) EMMCVPR 2015. LNCS, vol. 8932, pp. 126–140. Springer, Cham (2015). https://doi.org/10.1007/978-3-319-14612-6_10

15. Nocedal, J., Wright, S.J.: Numerical Optimization, 2nd edn. Springer, New York (2006). https://doi.org/10.1007/978-0-387-40065-5

16. Polfliet, M., et al.: Laplacian Eigenmaps for multimodal groupwise image registration. Medical Imaging 2017: Image Processing 10133: 101331N, International Society for Optics and Photonics (2017)

17. Sotiras, A., Davatzikos, C., Paragios, N.: Deformable medical image registration: a survey. IEEE Trans. Med. Imaging **32**(7), 1153–1190 (2013)

18. Sourbron, S.P., Buckley, D.L.: Classic models for dynamic contrast-enhanced MRI. NMR Biomed. **26**(8), 1004–1027 (2013)

19. Schmitt, O.: Die multimodale Architektonik des menschlichen Gehirns, Habilitation, Institute of Anatomy, Medical University of Lübeck (2001)

20. Streicher, J., Weninger, W.J., Müller, G.B.: External marker-based automatic congruencing: a new method of 3D reconstruction from serial sections. Anat. Rec. **248**(4), 583–602 (1997)

21. Tao, Q., et al.: Robust motion correction for myocardial T1 and extracellular volume mapping by principle component analysis-based groupwise image registration. J. Magn. Reson. Imaging **47**(5), 1397–1405 (2017). Wiley Online Library

22. Viola, P., Wells III, W.M.: Alignment by maximization of mutual information. Int. J. Comput. Vis. **24**(2), 137–154 (1997)

23. Wang, C.-W., Gosno, E.B., Li, Y.-S.: Fully automatic and robust 3D registration of serial-section microscopic images. Sci. Rep. **5**, 15051 (2015). Nature Publishing Group

24. Watrous, J.: Theory of Quantum Information, 2.3 Norms of operators, Lecture Notes, University of Waterloo (2011)

Semi-automated Processing of Real-Time CMR Scans for Left Ventricle Segmentation

Rahil Shahzad[1]([✉]), Martin Fasshauer[2], Boudewijn P. F. Lelieveldt[1,3], Joachim Lotz[2], and Rob van der Geest[1]

[1] Division of Image Processing (LKEB), Department of Radiology,
Leiden University Medical Center, Leiden, The Netherlands
r.shahzad@lumc.nl
[2] Institute for Diagnostic and Interventional Radiology,
University Medical Center Göttingen, Göttingen, Germany
[3] Intelligent Systems Department, Delft University of Technology,
Delft, The Netherlands

Abstract. We present a workflow for processing real-time cardiac MR (RT-CMR) scans for segmenting the left ventricle (LV) on short-axis slices (SAX). Our method is based on image registration, where the LV endocardium and epicardium are segmented by propagating a reference contour over all the frames of the RT-CMR SAX scans. Our method was evaluated on 19 subjects, the accuracy of the automatic LV endocardium and epicardium segmentation was compared to those defined manually. The proposed method obtained a dice similarity coefficient (DSC) of 0.94 and a mean surface-to-surface distance (MSD) measure of 0.89 ± 0.53 mm. Additionally, a number of automatically obtained clinical measures were compared to ground truth values. On average we obtained a Pearson's correlation coefficient (R) of 0.94 (0.99–0.74).

Keywords: Realtime-MR · Left ventricle · Segmentation
Registration · Semi-automatic

1 Introduction

Conventional Cardiac Magnetic Resonance (CMR) imaging interpolates a cardiac cycle from averaged data acquired over several heartbeats in order to evaluate cardiac function, these CMR scans require ECG triggering and breath-holding (for 10–15 s) [1]. Variations between heartbeats caused by arrhythmia blur the image due to this averaging. Also, some subjects are unable to hold their breaths for the duration of the scan which also result in blurred images. Moreover, beat-to-beat variations are believed to yield valuable information about early stages of heart failure as well as diseases to the heart muscle. To this end, a real-time CMR (RT-CMR) method has been developed that can achieve high-resolution imaging of a 2D slice at a high frame rate [2]. RT-CMR does not

© Springer International Publishing AG, part of Springer Nature 2018
S. Klein et al. (Eds.): WBIR 2018, LNCS 10883, pp. 57–66, 2018.
https://doi.org/10.1007/978-3-319-92258-4_6

require ECG triggering or breath-holding. Thus the sequence is able to acquire diagnostic quality images in patients with an irregular heart beat or for patients who have difficulty in holding their breaths [3].

In order to derive diagnostic information from the CMR scans a number of clinical measures have to be quantified. This is traditionally performed using (semi-)automatic image processing techniques on the conventional cine (2d + t) short-axis scans (SAX). Where the endocardium and the epicardium of the left ventricle (LV) is segmented from a number of slices extending from the apex to the base of the heart. The slices are segmented at the end-diastolic and the end-systolic cardiac phases to obtain the end-diastolic volume (EDV) and end-systolic volume (ESV), respectively. However, processing RT-CMR SAX scans using the traditional approach is unrealistic because of the sheer number of cardiac scans acquired for each SAX slice. Typically each RT-CMR SAX slice consists of 80–150 timepoints acquired over a number of cardiac cycles. Moreover, because no ECG triggering or breath-holding is used during acquisition, the location of the LV and the cardiac phase do not match between the SAX slices. Thus identifying the LV end-diastolic/systolic phases over the SAX slices is cumbersome.

The purpose of our study is to develop and evaluate a semi-automated method which is able to segment the LV endocardium and epicardium on all the acquired temporal frames and over multiple SAX slices using the RT-CMR scans. The LV segmentations are subsequently used to compute a number of clinically important measures such as the EDV, ESV, stroke volume (SV), ejection fraction (EF), and the myocardial mass.

2   Method

The proposed method consists of two main parts: (i) an image registration based approach for segmenting the LV endocardium and epicardium contours over all the acquired temporal frames, and (ii) a method that can identify the end diastolic and systolic timepoints from the segmented LV for every slice to compute the clinical measures.

2.1   Segmenting the Left Ventricle

An image registration based approach is used for delineating the LV endocardium and epicardium contours. Image registration based approaches [4] can be used to exploit the cyclic nature i.e. the continuous beating heart over multiple heart beats and model the deformation over the acquired cardiac scans. The RT-CMR short-axis cardiac data has two main motion components, the motion caused due to the beating heart, and the motion caused due to breathing.

To segment a region of interest (ROI) from the RT-CMR SAX slice, our method requires three steps: (i) all the timepoints from a SAX slice are simultaneously registered in a groupwise manner to compute forward transformations, (ii) to determine the coordinate mapping for each of the cardiac timepoints to the rest an inverse transformation is computed, and (iii) both the forward and

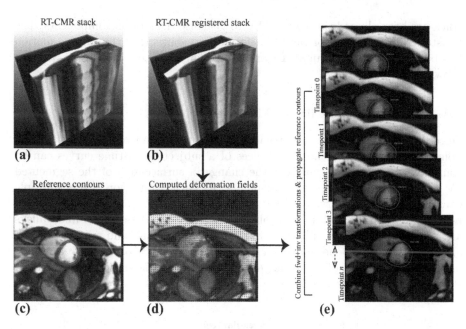

Fig. 1. Registration and contour propagation workflow. A single slice of RT-CMR image stacked over the time dimension (a). RT-CMR image stack after registration (b). Initialized endocardium (blue) and epicardium (red) contours on a single timepoint to be propagated (c). The computed deformation field for a random cardiac time point (d). The propagated contours over all the cardiac time points using the proposed workflow (e). (Color figure online)

the inverse transformations are combined such that a reference ROI defined on one timepoint can be transformed to the remaining timepoints. In our workflow the reference LV contours are manually defined in a single frame, usually on a frame where the LV can be clearly distinguished. Figure 1 shows a schematic of the registration approach.

The registration model used in this paper is based on the work of Metz *et al.* [5]. In brief, for the forward transformation this registration method incorporates spatiotemporal dimensions with the aim to minimize the change of voxel image intensity using a free-form B-spline transformation model. The method searches for the B-spline transformation that aligns all the cardiac timepoints to a mean frame by minimizing the variance of voxel intensity values over time. The registration method ensures a smooth deformation over the time dimension, which we expect from our cardiac data. An inverse transformation is computed in order to estimate the coordinate mapping from one timepoint to another. The inverse transformation is computed as a registration problem. For more details readers are referred to [5]. Using the obtained transformations reference contour(s) can then be propagated over all the timepoints for each of the SAX slices. Figure 1 shows a RT-CMR slice stacked along the time-dimension, the stack has been clipped through the LV to visualise the motion components. The registered image stack (forward transformation) shows that the cardiac motion has been accurately captured. Example of a few propagated contours are also shown.

2.2 Computing the Clinical Measures

Once the LV endocardium and epicardium have been segmented for all the timepoints and over all the short-axis slices of a subject. Area-time curves can be computed, these curves represent the change in surface-area of the segmented LV contour over the acquired timepoints. As each acquisition covers multiple cardiac cycles these curves display a number of peaks and valleys which correspond to diastolic and systolic phases respectively. These peaks and valleys are automatically detected by searching for local maxima's and minima's in the area-time curve. The end-diastolic and end-systolic area is obtained by computing the median value of the peaks and the valleys of the area-time curve for a slices. Figure 2 shows one such area-time curve.

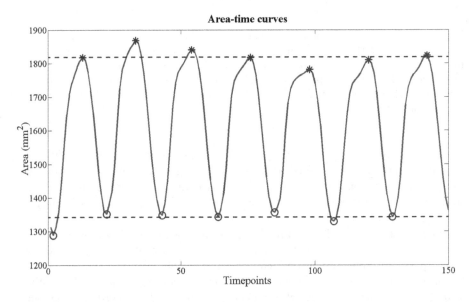

Fig. 2. Area-time curve for a random SAX slice. Dashed lines represent the median value of the peaks (*) and valleys (o).

The end diastolic volume (EDV) for a subject can be computed as:

$$EDV = \sum_{i=1}^{s} P_i * T,$$

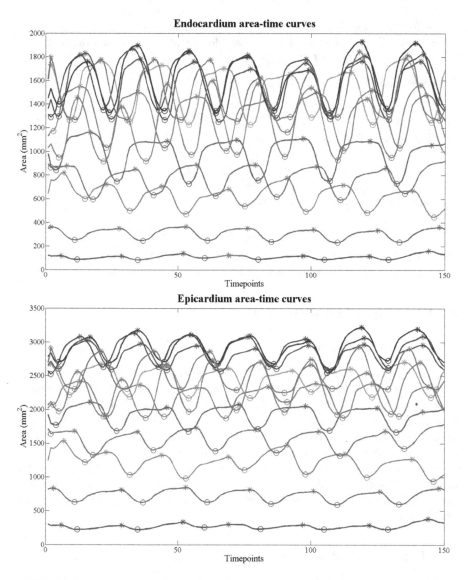

Fig. 3. Endocardium and epicardium area-time curves for a subject. Different colours correspond to different SAX slices, peaks and valleys are detected as '*' and 'o', respectively.

where i is the slice number, s is the maximum number of short-axis slices containing the LV, P is the median of the peak values for a slice and T is the slice thickness. The end systolic volume (ESV) is similarly obtained by summing over all the median values of the valleys (V). The EDV and ESV are obtained for the endocardium. Similarly the epicardial diastolic and systolic volumes can be obtained, by using the epicardial area-time curves. An example of the area-time curves for a subject is shown in Fig. 3. It should be noted that the peaks and the valleys (cardiac phases) of the curves do not align with each other, this is because the data is not ECG triggered.

Stroke volume (SV) is calculated as:

$$SV = EDV - ESV.$$

Ejection fraction (EF) is obtained as:

$$EF = \frac{SV}{EDV} \times 100\%.$$

Myocardial mass (Mass) is obtained as:

$$Mass = (EDV_{epi} - EDV_{endo}) * 1.05g,$$

where EDV_{epi} is the EDV of the epicardium and EDV_{endo} is the endocardial EDV, 1.05 is a constant which is used to obtain the mass in grams.

3   Experiments and Results

3.1   Data Acquisition

We retrospectively obtained 19 RT-CMR datasets of healthy subjects. These were acquired on Skyra 3T MRI scanner (Siemens Medical Solutions, Forchheim, Germany) at University Medical Center Göttingen (Germany). The scans have an in-plane resolution of 1.6×1.6 mm and a slice thickness of either 6 or 6.6 mm. Each of these subjects have either 80 or 150 timepoints with a temporal resolution of 33 ms. On a typical SAX scan the LV is covered by 11 slices.

Ground truth clinical measures were manually obtained for all 19 subjects, using MASS software (LUMC, Leiden, The Netherlands). An experienced user manually delineated the LV endocardium and epicardium on one diastolic and systolic phase.

3.2   Registration Parameters

All image registrations were performed using `elastix`, a publicly available registration software package [6]. Most of the registration parameters were optimized in our previous study (on cine CMR scans) [7]. Only minor changes had to be made to adapt for the RT-CMR scans. In short, registration was performed as follows. For both the forward and inverse registration a multi-resolution coarse-to-fine approach using four resolutions was used. Adaptive stochastic gradient descent was used for optimization [8]. The number of voxels randomly sampled in each iteration was set to 2000, and the number of iterations was also set to 2000. As a cost function "Variance Over Last Dimension" was used for forward registration and "Displacement Magnitude Penalty" for the inverse registration [5]. A B-spline grid was defined by control points with 10 mm separation in-plane

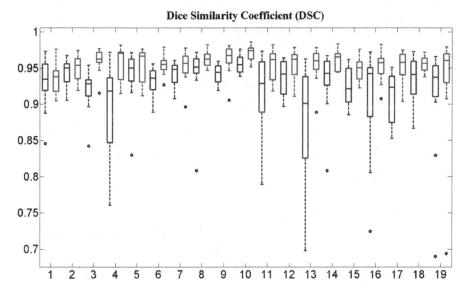

Fig. 4. Dice similarity coefficient for the LV endocardium (blue) and epicardium (red) contours over random multiple single slices for all 19 subject. (Color figure online)

and 1 mm in the time dimension. A powers-of-2 pyramid schedule for the grid was used over the 4 resolutions. The average registration time for a SAX slice is approximately 5 min on an desktop running Intel Xenon CPU 3.60 GHz and 16 GB RAM.

3.3 Results

To evaluate our method two experiments were carried out. In the first experiment, the quality of the LV segmentation was evaluated. This was done by comparing the dice similarity coefficient (DSC) and the mean surface-to-surface contour distance (MSD) between the automatically propagated contour and a manually defined contour. The manual contour was delineated by an independent user on a random timepoint on a few SAX slices (blinded to the segmentation results). In the second experiment, the clinical measures obtained using the proposed method were compared to the ground truth values. This was conducted by computing Pearson's correlation coefficient (R) and Bland-Altman analysis. Results show that the average DSC and MSD over all the subjects is 0.93 and 0.95 $\pm$ 0.55 mm, respectively for the endocardium, and 0.95 and 0.82 $\pm$ 0.52 mm for the epicardium contours. Figure 4 shows the DSC values for both the endocardium and the epicardium contours for each of the 19 subjects over multiple SAX slices. Table 1 shows the results for the clinical measures. Most of the measures have an R of 0.99 and narrow limits of agreement. The difference between the automatic method and the ground truth is not statistically significant. Figure 5 shows plots for three measures.

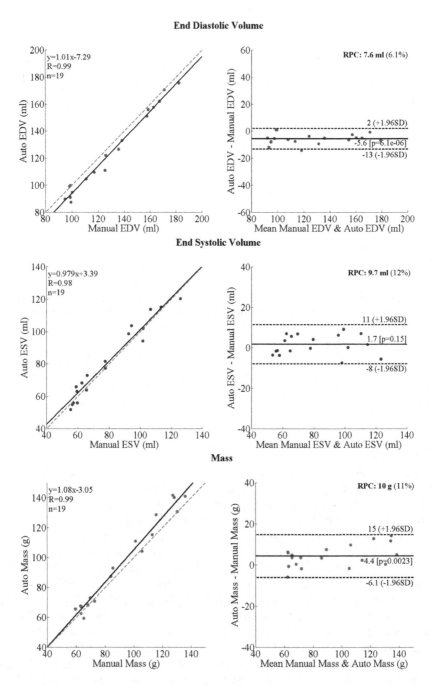

Fig. 5. Correlation and Bland-Altman plots for EDV, ESV and Mass. R is the Pearson's coefficient, n is the number of subjects and RCP is the reproducibility coefficient.

Table 1. Performance of the proposed method. R is the Pearson correlation coefficient. B-A is the Bland-Altman bias along with the 95% CI. Abs diff is the average absolute difference.

Measure	R	B-A (95% CI)	Abs diff
EDV (ml)	0.99	$-5.6(-13, 2)$	5.9 ± 3.5
ESV (ml)	0.98	$1.7(-8, 11)$	4.3 ± 2.7
SV (ml)	0.88	$-7.4(-17, 2)$	7.5 ± 4.6
EF (%)	0.74	$-4.3(-11, 2)$	4.6 ± 2.9
EDV_{epi} (ml)	0.99	$-1.5(-13, 10)$	4.5 ± 3.5
ESV_{epi} (ml)	0.99	$-8.0(-20, 4)$	8.3 ± 5.6
Mass (g)	0.99	$4.4(-6, 15)$	5.4 ± 4.3

4   Discussion and Conclusion

We present and evaluate a method for segmenting the LV from RT-CMR SAX scans. Results show good agreement with manual segmentation. Comparing the clinical measures showed excellent correlation with most of the ground truth measures. The values for stroke volume (SV) and ejection fraction (EF) were a bit low. This is mainly because the error accumulates over the end-diastolic (EDV) and end-systolic volumes (ESV). However, the myocardial mass has very good agreements.

The groupwise registration model used in this paper has advantages over the traditional pairwise registration approach as we do not have to provide a reference image during registration. This approach also avoids a bias towards a reference image and takes into account the intensity information of all images simultaneously. Moreover, this allows the user the freedom to choose any time-point for defining the reference LV contour used for propagation.

A drawback of our method is that we evaluated our method only on healthy subjects. But we do believe that our method would have a similar performance on subjects with arrhythmia. In the current work we have demonstrated the feasibility of using a semi-automated method to efficiently process RT-CMR scans to assess the cardiac function.

References

1. Manning, W.J., Pennell, D.J.: Cardiovascular Magnetic Resonance. Elsevier Health Sciences, Philadelphia (2010)
2. Zhang, S., Uecker, M., Voit, D., Merboldt, K.D., Frahm, J.: Real-time cardiovascular magnetic resonance at high temporal resolution: radial FLASH with nonlinear inverse reconstruction. J. Cardiovas. Magn. Reson. **12**(1), 39 (2010)
3. Uecker, M., Zhang, S., Voit, D., Karaus, A., Merboldt, K.D., Frahm, J.: Real-time MRI at a resolution of 20 ms. NMR in Biomed. **23**(8), 986–994 (2010)
4. Sotiras, A., Davatzikos, C., Paragios, N.: Deformable medical image registration: a survey. IEEE Trans. Med. Imaging **32**(7), 1153–1190 (2013)

5. Metz, C., Klein, S., Schaap, M., van Walsum, T., Niessen, W.J.: Nonrigid registration of dynamic medical imaging data using nD+t B-splines and a groupwise optimization approach. Med. Image Anal. **15**(2), 238–249 (2011)
6. Klein, S., Staring, M., Murphy, K., Viergever, M.A., Pluim, J.P.: Elastix: a toolbox for intensity-based medical image registration. IEEE Trans. Med. Imaging **29**(1), 196–205 (2010)
7. Shahzad, R., Tao, Q., Dzyubachyk, O., Staring, M., Lelieveldt, B.P., van der Geest, R.J.: Fully-automatic left ventricular segmentation from long-axis cardiac cine MR scans. Med. Image Anal. **39**, 44–55 (2017)
8. Klein, S., Pluim, J.P., Staring, M., Viergever, M.A.: Adaptive stochastic gradient descent optimisation for image registration. Int. J. Comput. Vis. **81**(3), 227 (2009)

Acceleration

Averaged Stochastic Optimization for Medical Image Registration Based on Variance Reduction

Wei Sun[1](✉), Dirk H. J. Poot[2], Xuan Yang[4], Wiro J. Niessen[2,3],
and Stefan Klein[1]

[1] Department of Neurology, Donders Institute for Brain, Cognition and Behaviour,
Donders Center for Medical Neuroscience, Radboud University Medical Center,
Nijmegen, The Netherlands
sunweidemail@gmail.com

[2] Biomedical Imaging Group Rotterdam, Erasmus MC, Rotterdam, The Netherlands

[3] Department of Image Science and Technology, Faculty of Applied Sciences,
Delft University of Technology, Delft, The Netherlands

[4] College of Computer Science and Software Engineering, Shenzhen University,
Shenzhen, Guangdong, China

Abstract. In image registration the optimal transformation parameters of a given transformation model are typically obtained by minimizing a cost function. Stochastic gradient descent (SGD) is an efficient optimization algorithm for image registration. In SGD optimization, stochastic approximations of the cost function derivative are used in each iteration to update the transformation parameters. The stochastic approximation error leads to large variance in the parameters. To enforce convergence nonetheless, SGD methods are typically implemented in combination with a gradually decreasing update step size. However, selecting a proper sequence of step sizes is a major challenge in practice. An alternative strategy in numerical optimization is to use a constant step size and enforce convergence by averaging the parameters obtained by SGD over several iterations. It was proven mathematically that the highest possible rate of convergence is achieved in this way. Inspired by this work, we propose an averaged SGD (Avg-SGD) method for efficient image registration. In the Avg-SGD approach, a constant step size is used, in combination with an exponentially weighted iterate averaging scheme. Experiments on 3D lung CT scans demonstrate the effectiveness of the Avg-SGD method in terms of convergence rate, accuracy and precision.

1 Introduction

To solve a registration problem, a cost function that measures the dissimilarity between images is usually defined, and then minimized by a numerical

---

W. Sun—This work was in part supported by the National Natural Science Foundation of China No. U1301251.

S. Klein et al. (Eds.): WBIR 2018, LNCS 10883, pp. 69–79, 2018.
https://doi.org/10.1007/978-3-319-92258-4_7

optimization routine. In [1], stochastic gradient descent (SGD) approach was implemented by using in each iteration a newly selected random subset of image data for calculation of the cost function gradient. So far, SGD approaches have been widely applied in many registration problems, e.g., [2–4]. In SGD optimization the issue of selecting a good sequence of step sizes γ is a major challenge in practice [5]. SGD methods are typically implemented in combination with a gradually decreasing step size. The selection of γ is critical for the performance of the optimization process. If the step size γ is chosen too small, the minimizing process of the cost function will be too slow and easily get stuck at an early stage. If γ is selected too large, the noise during the stochastic optimization will become too large and the reliability of the optimization cannot be guaranteed. In both cases, the convergence rates of optimization are not optimal. To estimate γ automatically in image registration problems, an adaptive stochastic gradient descent (ASGD) optimizer was proposed in [6]. In the ASGD method, an image-driven mechanism is used to predict a reasonable value of γ, which satisfies several theoretical conditions for convergence. However, the ASGD optimizer has a relatively high computation cost during the estimation process when the number of transformation parameters becomes high. To tackle this issue, a fast ASGD optimizer was proposed in [7]. Although the ASGD method provides a reasonable choice of γ, it does not claim to achieve an optimal rate of convergence.

The convergence rate of SGD can be accelerated by using the second-order information (i.e., Hessian matrix) of the cost function. When the second-order information is adopted, the former scalar γ becomes a matrix which is employed to control the step size according to the curvature of the optimization landscape. Because the second-order information is not known in advance, various methods for predicting the Hessian matrix were proposed in [8]. However, the computational cost of determining the full Hessian matrix is usually too high to maintain. Therefore, different approaches for estimating an approximated Hessian matrix were proposed in [9]. However, those approximated estimations cannot guarantee a convergence rate which is as good as when using the full Hessian matrix in practice [10].

An alternative strategy to accelerate the convergence rate was proposed by Polyak and Juditsky [11]. They proposed to average the iterates of a SGD optimization, and proved that the averaged sequence of the estimated parameters converges in an optimal rate, which is as good as full second-order SGD. We refer to this method as Avg-SGD. With this approach, we may use a larger than usual step size γ and let the averaging take care of the increased noise effects that are due to the larger step size. In this way we can substantially improve the overall convergence speed and make the choice of γ less critical. Compared with the second-order SGD, the averaging technique is easy to implement and more attractive in practice.

In this paper we investigate the potential of the Avg-SGD method for image registration. In theoretical analyses, it is typically assumed that the iteration number $k \to \infty$ [5]. However, this assumption is impractical for image registration where we only have limited computation time. Given finite k, it is preferable to skip or alleviate the effect of iterates in the early phase of optimization because the estimated transformation parameters may change dramatically. In this research, we present an exponential Avg-SGD method where the effect of the early iterations is exponentially decreased, avoiding the need to set a hard threshold k_0 for the commence of averaging. We compared the new Avg-SGD method with the state-of-the-art ASGD optimizer in the experiments on 3D real imaging data with nonrigid registration.

2 Method

2.1 Stochastic Optimization for Image Registration

Let $F(\boldsymbol{x}) : \Omega_F \subset \mathbb{R}^D \to \mathbb{R}$ and $M(\boldsymbol{x}) : \Omega_M \subset \mathbb{R}^D \to \mathbb{R}$ denote the D-dimensional fixed and moving images where $\boldsymbol{x}$ represents an image coordinate, and Ω_F and Ω_M are the fixed and moving image domains, respectively. Suppose $\mathbf{T}(\boldsymbol{\mu}, \boldsymbol{x}) : \mathbb{R}^P \times \Omega_F \to \Omega_M$ is a coordinate transformation where $\boldsymbol{\mu} \in \mathbb{R}^P$ represents the vector of transformation parameters. $\mathbf{T}(\boldsymbol{\mu}, \boldsymbol{x})$ could be a translation, rigid, affine or nonrigid (e.g., B-spline) transformation model. Then, the registration problem is defined as:

$$\hat{\boldsymbol{\mu}} = \arg \min_{\boldsymbol{\mu}} \mathcal{C}\left(\boldsymbol{\mu}, \Omega_F\right), \tag{1}$$

where $\mathcal{C}(\boldsymbol{\mu}, \Omega_F)$ calculates the dissimilarity between the original fixed image $F(\boldsymbol{x})$ and the deformed moving image $M(\mathbf{T}(\boldsymbol{\mu}, \boldsymbol{x}))$ on the domain $\boldsymbol{x} \in \Omega_F$. Examples of $\mathcal{C}$ are mutual information [12], the sum of squared differences (SSD), and normalized correlation coefficient. For instance, the cost function $\mathcal{C}$ of SSD is defined as:

$$\mathcal{C}\left(\boldsymbol{\mu}, \Omega_F\right) = \frac{1}{|\Omega_F|} \sum_{\boldsymbol{x}_i \in \Omega_F} \left(F(\boldsymbol{x}_i) - M\left(\mathbf{T}(\boldsymbol{\mu}, \boldsymbol{x}_i)\right)\right)^2. \tag{2}$$

In image registration, an iterative optimization strategy is applied to solve Eq. (1) and determine the optimal set of parameters $\hat{\boldsymbol{\mu}}$. In the evaluation of different optimizers [1], the SGD optimizer turned out to be a competitive alternative to deterministic algorithms in nonrigid registration problems. SGD optimization is based on the following iterative update strategy:

$$\boldsymbol{\mu}_{k+1} = \boldsymbol{\mu}_k - \gamma_k \tilde{\boldsymbol{g}}_k, \quad k = 0, 1, 2 \ldots K, \tag{3}$$

where $\tilde{\boldsymbol{g}}_k$ represents a stochastic approximation of the cost function derivative $\partial \mathcal{C} / \partial \boldsymbol{\mu}$, evaluated at the current estimated transformation parameters $\boldsymbol{\mu}_k$, and γ_k is a scalar gain factor that controls the step size along $\tilde{\boldsymbol{g}}_k$.

2.2 Averaged Stochastic Gradient Descent (Avg-SGD)

Let us define

$$\lim_{k \to \infty} \boldsymbol{\mu}_k = \boldsymbol{\mu}^*. \tag{4}$$

The asymptotic normality under certain assumptions of the rate of convergence of SGD can be defined as [6]:

$$\sqrt{k}(\boldsymbol{\mu}_k - \boldsymbol{\mu}^*) \xrightarrow{d} \mathcal{N}(\mathbf{0}, \boldsymbol{V}), \tag{5}$$

where $\xrightarrow{d}$ represents the convergence in distribution as $k \to \infty$, and $\mathcal{N}(\mathbf{0}, \boldsymbol{V})$ is a multivariate normal distribution with mean $\mathbf{0}$ and covariance matrix $\boldsymbol{V}$.

To accelerate the convergence of stochastic optimization, Polyak and Juditsky [11] and Ruppert [13] proposed to average the trajectory of stochastic optimization. In contrast to other accelerating techniques (e.g., second-order SGD), the averaging technique is simple and requires no prior information about the cost function. The original Polyak averaging can be formulated as:

$$\bar{\boldsymbol{\mu}}_k = \frac{1}{k+1} \sum_{i=0}^{k} \boldsymbol{\mu}_i, \tag{6}$$

where $\bar{\boldsymbol{\mu}}_k$ is the sequence of averaged parameters. It is worth noting that this iterate averaging process does not interfere with the original SGD algorithm; the estimates $\boldsymbol{\mu}_k$ are unaffected by $\bar{\boldsymbol{\mu}}_k$. The basic idea is that $\bar{\boldsymbol{\mu}}_k$ converges faster to $\boldsymbol{\mu}^*$ than $\boldsymbol{\mu}_k$ does. In [11], Polyak and Juditsky presented a proof that $\bar{\boldsymbol{\mu}}_k$ converges to $\boldsymbol{\mu}^*$ as good as the full second-order algorithm. In later work [14], Yin showed that

$$\sqrt{k}(\bar{\boldsymbol{\mu}}_k - \boldsymbol{\mu}^*) \xrightarrow{d} \mathcal{N}(\mathbf{0}, \bar{\boldsymbol{V}}), \tag{7}$$

where $\bar{\boldsymbol{V}}$ is the smallest possible covariance matrix when an asymptotically optimal matrix-valued step size (e.g., second-order SGD) is adopted.

If $\gamma_k \to 0$ slower than $O(1/k)$, Kushner and Yin extended the averaging theory to a window definition [5]:

$$\bar{\boldsymbol{\mu}}_k^{win} = \frac{\gamma_k}{\tau} \sum_{i=k-\tau/\gamma_k+1}^{k} \boldsymbol{\mu}_i, \tag{8}$$

where $k \geq \tau/\gamma_k - 1$ and the number of iterates in the window of averaging is $\tau/\gamma_k = o(k)$ for arbitrary real $\tau > 0$. They proved that

$$(\bar{\boldsymbol{\mu}}_k^{win} - \boldsymbol{\mu}^*) \xrightarrow{d} \mathcal{N}(\mathbf{0}, \frac{\gamma_k \bar{\boldsymbol{V}}}{\tau}). \tag{9}$$

Equation (9) shows that the covariance matrix $\bar{\boldsymbol{V}}$ can be reduced proportionally to the size of averaging window τ/γ_k. In [5], they confirmed that this desirable property of averaging holds both for constant and decreasing step size γ_k.

In practice, we only have a finite number of iterations K which is different from the theoretical analysis under the assumption $k \to \infty$. Because $\boldsymbol{\mu}_i$ may change substantially in the initial phase of optimization, it would be preferable to skip or alleviate the effect of first k_0 iterations in Eq. (6). One easy way is to skip the iterations before k_0, and only the iterates from k_0 to k are averaged to compute $\bar{\boldsymbol{\mu}}_k^{post}$. However, there is no prior information to properly choose k_0 for a practical problem. If k_0 is too small, the 'premature' $\boldsymbol{\mu}_i$ where $i \leq k_0$ could be involved in the averaging calculation. If k_0 is too large, the number of averaged iterates will become too low to achieve substantial acceleration of convergence.

To remedy the issue of choosing k_0, we define an *exponential* moving average:

$$\bar{\boldsymbol{\mu}}_{k+1}^{ex} = (1 - \epsilon)\bar{\boldsymbol{\mu}}_k^{ex} + \epsilon\boldsymbol{\mu}_{k+1} = (1 - \epsilon)^{k+1}\boldsymbol{\mu}_0 + \epsilon\sum_{j=1}^{k+1}(1 - \epsilon)^{k+1-j}\boldsymbol{\mu}_j, \qquad (10)$$

where $0 < \epsilon < 1$ and $\bar{\boldsymbol{\mu}}_0^{ex} = \boldsymbol{\mu}_0$. In this exponential averaging method, the influence of previous iterates is decreased exponentially. In this way, we avoid the need to set a hard threshold k_0. The influence of initial iterations is gradually decayed. The weighing factor ϵ needs to be set by the user. In this work, we fixed ϵ to a constant parameter for all experiments.

Note that for the choice $\epsilon = 1/(k + 2)$, Eq. (10) boils down to a recursive formulation of the original Polyak averaging method (Eq. (6)).

Table 1. Summary of registration methods.

Method	Step size (γ)	Optimization
SGD-constant	Constant	SGD
SGD-adaptive	Adaptively decreasing	SGD
Avg-constant	Constant	Avg-SGD
Avg-adaptive	Adaptively decreasing	Avg-SGD

2.3 Step Size Selection

The use of Avg-SGD may allow us to use a constant step size γ instead of a decaying step size, which may benefit the convergence rate in non-asymptotic settings. The increased noise on $\boldsymbol{\mu}_k$ due to the large step sizes in later iterations could be attenuated by the averaging process in the Avg-SGD method. In this work, we will therefore compare different step size selection schemes in combination with the Avg-SGD and conventional SGD approaches. Table 1 summarizes the registration methods evaluated in this work. In Table 1, the SGD-constant method represents the ordinary SGD optimizer using constant γ. The SGD-adaptive method is the standard ASGD optimizer equipped with adaptively decreasing γ in [6]. The Avg-constant method represents the proposed Avg-SGD approach using constant γ. The Avg-adaptive approach is the Avg-SGD method combined with the adaptively decreasing γ. The initial step sizes of all methods are the same and calculated as described in [6].

3   Experiments

As a generic technique, the Avg-SGD approach can in principle be used in combination with any transformation model and similarity metric. In this work, we evaluated the Avg-SGD method in the setting of nonrigid B-spline transformation model using SSD metrics for 3D lung CT registration problem. All methods were implemented as part of the open source image registration package elastix [15]. The number of random samples S was set to 2000. The number of iterations K of the optimizer was set to 2000. For the Avg-SGD in Eq. (10), we fixed $\epsilon = 0.01$ in all experiments.

To investigate the performance on different distortion levels, we used a multilevel optimization, in which the transformation parameters $\hat{\mu}$ estimated at level l were used to initialize μ_0 at level $l + 1$. For this purpose, we used the result $\hat{\mu} = \mu_K$ obtained by the conventional SGD-adaptive method, to ensure that in each level all methods start from the same point μ_0. No image blurring was performed. Two levels were used for the nonrigid registration experiments. The B-spline control point spacing η was set to 64 and 32 mm in the two levels, respectively.

3.1   Evaluation Measures

To quantify different aspects of convergence behavior, we use three measures: accuracy curves, reproducibility curves, and fluctuation.

Let $\Gamma(k)$ represent registration accuracy as a function of the iteration number k. We compute the mean of $\Gamma(k)$ over multiple registration cases, and plot this mean as a function of k, to obtain accuracy curves. The reproducibility measure assesses the change of the registration accuracy caused by intrinsic randomness of SGD optimization. To quantify this, the registrations were repeated with $R = 20$ random seeds. The random seed affects the selection of the random subsets $\widetilde{\Omega}_F^k$ which represents the random samples $\widetilde{\Omega}_F$ at iteration k. The standard deviation of registration accuracy was calculated over those seeds to measure the reproducibility of each method. Thus, we can define the reproducibility as: $\text{Std}(\Gamma_r(k))$ with $\Gamma_r(k)$ the accuracy at iteration k using random seed r. In the experiments, the reproducibility is evaluated at multiple iterations k and is plotted as a function of k, in order to obtain reproducibility curves.

The fluctuation of the accuracy curve over the last 100 iterations was computed to assess the variability of the registration result near the end of optimization procedure. Large fluctuation of $\Gamma(k)$ in the final iterations would indicate the optimization has not fully converged yet. The second-order derivative of the curve was adopted to measure the fluctuation. The second-order derivative at iteration k can be approximated by finite difference:

$$\Gamma''(k) \approx \Gamma(k + 1) - 2\Gamma(k) + \Gamma(k - 1), \tag{11}$$

where $\Gamma(k)$ represents the registration accuracy at iteration k. For each test case, we calculate the root mean square of these second-order derivatives over the last 100 iterations, and we summarize the results of all test cases using box plots.

3.2   Nonrigid Registration on 3D Lung CT

The publicly available DIR-Lab 3D chest CT data set facilitates a rigorous and objective assessment of the spatial accuracy of registration methods [16]. The DIR-Lab data set contains 10 pairs of scans with 300 manually annotated landmarks on the lungs, which allows us to evaluate the registration accuracy. The voxel sizes and dimensions of these scans are around $1.0 \times 1.0 \times 2.5$ mm and around $256 \times 256 \times 110$ voxels. To focus on the lung region, lung masks were created to restrict the registration. The masks were created by thresholding, 3D-6-neighborhood connected component analysis, and morphological closing operation using a spherical kernel with a diameter of 9 voxels. In the experiments, the exhale phase (moving image) was registered to the inhale phase (fixed image). The mean of target registration errors (TRE), which measure the distances between the transformed and ground truth landmarks, was used to measure the registration accuracy Γ. Here, each test was repeated with 20 random seeds. Therefore, there are in total 10×20 test cases for 10 patients over 20 random seeds.

4   Results

Figure 1 shows the results of candidate approaches using two-level registration on lung CT data. Figures 1(a) and (c) present the mean of $\Gamma(k)$ over 10×20 registration cases, at each iteration $k = 0, 100, 200, \ldots K$ for the first and second registration levels, respectively. As shown in Fig. 1(a) the methods using constant γ converged faster than the approaches using adaptively decreasing γ at the first registration level. It can also be found that the SGD-constant and Avg-constant method obtained similar final accuracy. At the second registration level (Fig. 1(c)), the methods using constant γ still outperformed the approaches using adaptively decreasing γ. In addition, the proposed Avg-constant method achieved a better convergence rate than the SGD-constant approach.

Table 2. Registration accuracy (mm) on lung CT data using B-spline transformation.

	SGD-constant	SGD-adaptive	Avg-constant	Avg-adaptive
Level 1	1.66 ± 0.37	1.92 ± 0.77	$\mathbf{1.65 \pm 0.32}$	1.92 ± 0.78
Level 2	1.45 ± 0.28	1.46 ± 0.35	$\mathbf{1.43 \pm 0.28}$	1.46 ± 0.35

The results of final registration accuracy achieved by candidate approaches at each registration level are presented in Table 2. It can be observed that the

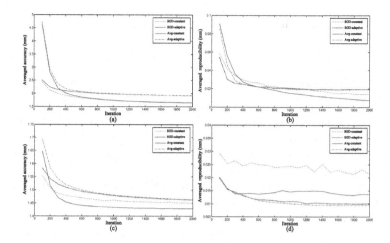

Fig. 1. Convergence curve and reproducibility curves of registration methods on lung CT data using B-spline transformation. (a) and (c) averaged convergence curves on from the first to the second registration levels over 10×20 test cases; (b) and (d) averaged reproducibility curves from the first to the second registration levels over 10×20 test cases.

proposed Avg-constant method constantly generated the best registration accuracy at each level. In comparison with the previous research on the same data [17], the averaged registration accuracy reported in Table 2 is better.

Figures 1(b) and (d) show the reproducibility $\text{Std}(\Gamma_r(k))$ over 20 random seeds. The reproducibilities are averaged over 10 patients. As shown in Fig. 1(b), the final values of $\text{Std}(\Gamma_r(k))$ of the SGD-constant and Avg-constant approaches are better than the methods using adaptively decreasing γ. It can be noticed that the Avg-constant method achieved the best reproducibility. At the second registration level (Fig. 1(d)), the SGD-constant method was the least reproducible among all methods. In contrast, the reproducibility was improved by using the Avg-constant method.

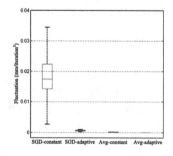

Fig. 2. Degrees of fluctuations of registration methods on lung CT data.

Figure 2 shows the degree of fluctuation at the final registration level on lung data. It can be observed that the SGD-constant method produced the largest fluctuation among all methods. However, the proposed Avg-constant approach reduced the fluctuation substantially.

5 Discussion

We proposed the Avg-SGD optimization method for image registration. The Avg-SGD method uses a constant instead of a decreasing step size γ, in order to accelerate optimization. The averaging process of the Avg-SGD approach compensates for the increased noise due to constant γ. The performance of the Avg-SGD method was evaluated in comparison to the state-of-the-art ASGD optimizer. The improvements in registration accuracy, registration reproducibility and fluctuation of the convergence curve prove the effectiveness of the Avg-SGD method.

For large initial deformation, both the SGD-constant and Avg-constant methods achieved faster convergence rate than the approaches using adaptively decreasing γ. However, the constant γ resulted in large fluctuations around the optimum and thus lower reproducibility of the final solution obtained by the SGD-constant approach. The proposed Avg-SGD approach compensates for the fluctuations caused by constant γ, which was confirmed by the improved reproducibility curves. Compared with the methods using constant γ, the approaches using adaptively decreasing γ even obtained lower reproducibility. The reason is that these methods did not really converge yet at $k = K$, which causes a higher variation over different random seeds.

For small initial deformation, the noise caused by the constant γ has significant influence on the SGD method. The better convergence rate was still preserved by using the new Avg-SGD method. The reproducibility of the result in case of small initial deformation proves that the Avg-SGD method can effectively reduce the noise effect due to constant γ.

The fluctuation of the convergence curve was also evaluated to measure registration precision. The variation of the accuracy over iterations is reflected by the fluctuation measure. The boxplots (Fig. 2) clearly showed that the SGD-constant method results in large fluctuations in the final iterations. This is exactly the reason why SGD methods are usually implemented with decreasing step sizes; due to the stochastic noise on the gradients $\tilde{g}_k$ convergence needs to be enforced in some way. To achieve this, commonly, the step size is decreased with increasing iteration number k. Indeed, the SGD-adaptive method resulted in low fluctuation values. In this work, the Avg-SGD method proved to be another effective way to dampen the fluctuations and enforce convergence, eliminating the need to decrease the step size.

Regarding the computation time, the Avg-SGD approach was implemented in a recursive manner. During the optimization, only one set of averaged transformation parameters needs to be stored. To update the averaged parameters we only need simple vector operations. Therefore, the additional computational cost raised by the Avg-SGD method is trivial in practice.

6 Conclusion

We developed the Avg-SGD optimization method for image registration. The proposed approach compensates for the stochastic noise inherent to SGD by averaging over iterations. Thanks to the iterative averaging, large step sizes can be maintained throughout the entire optimization process, resulting in accelerated convergence while preserving the registration precision. The improved registration results demonstrate the effectiveness of the Avg-SGD method.

References

1. Klein, S., Staring, M., Pluim, J.P.W.: Evaluation of optimization methods for nonrigid medical image registration using mutual information and B-splines. IEEE Trans. Image Process. **16**(12), 2879–2890 (2007)
2. Viola, P., Wells III, W.M.: Alignment by maximization of mutual information. Int. J. Comput. Vis. **24**(2), 137–154 (1997)
3. Sun, W., Poot, D.H., Smal, I., Yang, X., Niessen, W.J., Klein, S.: Stochastic optimization with randomized smoothing for image registration. Med. Image Anal. **35**, 146–158 (2017)
4. Sun, W., Niessen, W.J., Klein, S.: Randomly perturbed B-splines for nonrigid image registration. IEEE Trans. Pattern Anal. Mach. Intell. **39**(7), 1401–1413 (2017)
5. Kushner, H.J., Yin, G.: Stochastic Approximation and Recursive Algorithms and Applications, vol. 35. Springer, New York (2003). https://doi.org/10.1007/b97441
6. Klein, S., Pluim, J.P.W., Staring, M., Viergever, M.A.: Adaptive stochastic gradient descent optimisation for image registration. Int. J. Comput. Vis. **81**(3), 227–239 (2009)
7. Qiao, Y., van Lew, B., Lelieveldt, B.P., Staring, M.: Fast automatic step size estimation for gradient descent optimization of image registration. IEEE Trans. Med. Imaging **35**(2), 391–403 (2016)
8. Bottou, L., Le Cun, Y.: On-line learning for very large data sets. Appl. Stoch. Models. Bus. Ind. **21**(2), 137–151 (2005)
9. Bordes, A., Bottou, L., Gallinari, P.: SGD-QN: careful quasi-Newton stochastic gradient descent. J. Mach. Learn. Res. **10**, 1737–1754 (2009)
10. Xu, W.: Towards optimal one pass large scale learning with averaged stochastic gradient descent. arXiv preprint arXiv:1107.2490 (2011)
11. Polyak, B.T., Juditsky, A.B.: Acceleration of stochastic approximation by averaging. SIAM J. Control Optim. **30**(4), 838–855 (1992)
12. Maes, F., Collignon, A., Vandermeulen, D., Marchal, G., Suetens, P.: Multimodality image registration by maximization of mutual information. IEEE Trans. Med. Imaging **16**(2), 187–198 (1997)
13. Ruppert, D.: Efficient estimations from a slowly convergent Robbins-Monro process. Technical report, Cornell University Operations Research and Industrial Engineering (1988)
14. Yin, G.: Stochastic approximation via averaging: the Polyak's approach revisited. In: Pflug, G., Dieter, U. (eds.) Simulation and Optimization. Lecture Notes in Economics and Mathematical Systems, vol. 374, pp. 119–134. Springer, Heidelberg (1992). https://doi.org/10.1007/978-3-642-48914-3_9

15. Klein, S., Staring, M., Murphy, K., Viergever, M.A., Pluim, J.P.W.: Elastix: a toolbox for intensity-based medical image registration. IEEE Trans. Med. Imaging **29**(1), 196–205 (2010)
16. Castillo, R., Castillo, E., Guerra, R., Johnson, V., McPhail, T., Garg, A., Guerrero, T.: A framework for evaluation of deformable image registration spatial accuracy using large landmark point sets. Phys. Med. Biol. **54**(7), 1849–1870 (2009)
17. Papież, B.W., Heinrich, M.P., Fehrenbach, J., Risser, L., Schnabel, J.A.: An implicit sliding-motion preserving regularisation via bilateral filtering for deformable image registration. Med. Image Anal. **18**(8), 1299–1311 (2014)

Applications and Evaluation

Registration Evaluation by De-enhancing CT Images

Manh Ha Luu[1,2], Hassan Boulkhrif[3], Adriaan Moelker[3],
and Theo van Walsum[1(✉)]

[1] Biomedical Imaging Group Rotterdam Departments of Radiology & Nuclear
Medicine and Medical Informatics, Erasmus MC – University Medical Center
Rotterdam, Rotterdam, The Netherlands
t.vanwalsum@erasmusmc.nl
[2] AVITECH – University of Technology and Engineering, VNU, Hanoi, Vietnam
[3] Department of Radiology & Nuclear Medicine, Erasmus MC – University Medical
Center Rotterdam, Rotterdam, The Netherlands

Abstract. Image registration is relevant for many medical procedures.
For CT-guided ablation procedures, integrating the lesion location from
diagnostic contrast-enhanced CT (CECT) images in interventional CT
images may provide better guidance for the interventional radiologist.
The main requirement for such methods is to accurately align the lesion
location. This, in general, can not be measured, and often surrogates are
used for the assessment. In this work, we present a method that permits
the assessment of the accuracy of the lesion localization, i.e. assessing the
value that is relevant for clinical practice. To this end, we developed a
method that virtually removes the contrast agent from an interventional
CT image, use this image for the registration, and use the original CECT
image for the assessment. For the experimental evaluation, imaging data
of 20 subjects (33 lesions) were used, and the registration accuracy of a
publicly available registration method was assessed using this method.

1   Introduction

Image guided minimally invasive interventions may benefit from registration to
align preoperative information (images, planning) with the patient during the
intervention.

The clinical context of this manuscript deals with percutaneous CT-guided
ablations of liver tumors. This is a minimally invasive intervention where a needle is introduced through the skin, such that the needle tip is at the lesion center,
after which energy (radiofrequency or micro wave) is applied to locally heat the
lesion and kill its cells. Correct needle placement is of paramount importance,
as incorrect placement may lead to partial ablation and recurrence of the lesion
and it may lead to excessive destruction of healthy tissue. Therefore, this intervention is performed using image guidance: an interventional modality is used
to visualize the needle and the lesion. Generally, ultrasound, being a safe and
real-time modality, is being used for guidance, but not all lesions show sufficient

contrast in ultrasound. Therefore, CT imaging is also used as an interventional modality for percutaneous ablations.

In CT-guidance first an unenhanced image is acquired, which serves as an overview to plan the needle introduction. Subsequently, a needle is advanced, with regular checks done by obtaining a CT image with the needle in place. After the ablation, a CT scan with contrast is being made to assess the treatment.

Lesion localization in the initial unenhanced CT image may be difficult, as many lesions are only visible on contrast-enhanced CT (CECT) images. Contrast agent is toxic, and can be used only once during an intervention, and is preferably used to assess the treatment. However, a contrast-enhanced diagnostic scan, showing the lesion and possibly other structures, is commonly available. Therefore, interventionalists use a "mental mapping" approach, combining the information from the diagnostic scan and the interventional scan, to map the lesion location.

The latter task may be performed by a registration algorithm as well, and several groups have investigated registration approaches that enable the anatomical alignment of the liver in two CT scans. A crucial issue is the final Target Registration Error (TRE) for these methods. Assessment of registration accuracy was considered an important issue ten years ago [1], and it still is today. Rohlfing [2] demonstrated, be it in a rather artificial example that overlap and similarity metrics are not always good predictors of registration accuracy. Still, TRE is often not known and reported: most of the methods have been evaluated by using surrogate measures such as Dice and Mean Surface Distance (MSD) or Hausdorff Distance (HD) over the liver surface [3–7]. The choice of these metrics is caused by the lack of a reference standard for the lesion location in the unenhanced image, an issue that is occurring more often in registration evaluation. Interesting approaches are the assessment of landmarks, such as is done in the lung CT challenges, and for which automated approaches have been presented [8]. However, anatomical landmarks, because of their appearance in the images, may align better than regions without a clear structure, such as is the case in our application. Others have proposed to simulate deformations [9], which provides a good ground truth for the assessment of the deformation field.

For clinical assessment, however, we are interested in assessing the target registration error, and also investigating how that relates metrics such as mean surface distance.

Purpose of this paper therefore is to develop and evaluate a method that permits to assess the target registration accuracy for this liver registration problem. The main contributions are a method to virtually de-enhance a CECT scan, and the application of this method in assessing the TRE of an existing registration method. In the following, we first detail the background and method of the virtual de-enhancement contrast, and next we describe the experiments and the results, which are followed by a discussion and conclusion.

2 Method

The key idea behind the method is to use a contrast-enhanced interventional scan for the evaluation. This scan contains the spatial information of the lesion, and this information can serve as the ground truth. To prevent the registration algorithm to be guided by the effects of contrast-enhancement (vessel visibility, hyper- or hypointense lesions), the effect of the contrast agent is removed from the image by a semi-automatic post-processing method. The resulting so-called virtual un-enhanced CT (VUCT) image is subsequently used by the registration approach, see Fig. 1. In this way, the registration cannot utilize the contrast agent effects, thus mimicking the clinical target situation, while there is a good reference standard for measuring the target registration error.

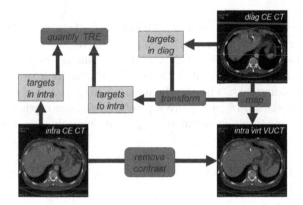

Fig. 1. Overall process of registration evaluation: the interventional CECT image (bottom left) is de-enhanced, after which this virtually unenhanced image is used in the registration. The lesion center obtained by transforming this position from the diagnostic scan to the interventional scan after registration is compared to the lesion center in the original interventional scan, which was manually obtained.

In the following, each of the steps of the de-enhancement are explained in more detail, see also Fig. 2.

2.1 Hyperintense Lesions and Vessels

As a prerequisite of the method, a segmentation of the liver is required. Whereas several methods for automated liver segmentation are available, we used a manual segmentation for this process. For a given image I we denote the liver mask with M_l. Furthermore, we compute the statistics of the pixel intensities of the liver, μ_l and σ_l.

Structures that are contrast-enhanced in the liver are vessels (mainly the veins, as the images are generally portal-venous scans) and the lesion. There may be other hyper-intense structures in the liver, that are not the result of the

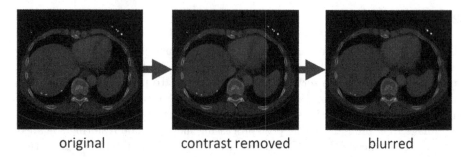

original   contrast removed   blurred

Fig. 2. De-enhancement process: left the original CECT, middle the vessels and the tumor pixels are filled with intensity values in the range of the liver parenchyma, right a blurred version of the middle one.

contrast enhancement, such as calcifications or surgical clips. As these structures may guide the registration process, we do not want to remove these. Generally, these structures are of higher intensity then the contrast-enhanced structures. Therefore, we use a thresholding with two thresholds to select the candidate pixels for de-enhancement. The thresholds are defined in terms of the mean μ_l and standard deviation σ_l of the liver pixels. Thus, the mask containing hyperintense voxels to be de-enhanced, M_{high}, is determined as follows (with p a pixel):

$$M_{high}(p) = \begin{cases} 1 & \text{if } \mu_l + \alpha_1 * \sigma_l < I(p) < \mu_l + \beta_1 * \sigma_l \text{ and } M_l(p) = 1 \\ 0 & \text{else} \end{cases} , \quad (1)$$

where α_1 and β_1 are parameters that are set per patient. In the end, these voxels' values will be replaced with random gaussian values determined by the distribution of the normal liver values, yielding the image I_{high}:

$$I_{high}(p) = \begin{cases} N(\mu_l + \alpha_2 * \sigma_l, \beta_2 * \sigma_l) & \text{if } M_{high}(p) = 1 \\ 0 & \text{else} \end{cases} , \quad (2)$$

where α_2 and β_2 are parameters to be set per image.

2.2 Hypointense Lesions

For the hypointense lesions, a similar strategy is followed. However, intensity based thresholding such as done for the hyperintense lesions is not feasible, as there are other low intensity structures with similar intensity that need to be retained. Therefore, hypointense lesions are segmented manually, and subsequently a similar procedure is followed to construct M_{low} and I_{low} as for the hyperintense lesions.

2.3   Granularity and Borders

The initial non-enhanced image I_{VU-0} is obtained by a masked combination of the three images:

$$I_{VU-0} = I \cdot (\text{not}(M_{high}(or)M_{low})) + I_{high} \cdot M_{high} + I_{low} \cdot M_{low}. \qquad (3)$$

In I_{VU-0}, the lesions and the vessels may still be visible, because of the difference in granularity. Additionally, the borders between the liver pixels and the de-enhanced regions are still clear. To address the granularity issue, I_{VU-0} is Gaussian blurred with a sigma of σ_g, yielding I'_{VU-0}, which is subsequently used to replace the low and high intensity voxels:

$$I_{VU-1} = I \cdot (\text{not}(M_{high}(or)M_{low})) + I'_{VU-0} \cdot (M_{high}\text{or}M_{low}) \qquad (4)$$

Subsequently, a similar blurring approach is applied to hide the borders between the liver pixels and the replaced pixels, giving the final virtually unenhanced image I_{VU}:

$$I_{VU} = I \cdot \text{not}(M_l) + I'_{VU-1} \cdot M_l \qquad (5)$$

2.4   Parameter Settings

The method has several parameter settings: the intensity threshold parameters (two for hyperintense and two for hypointense lesions), and the parameters for the distribution replacing the intensities (again two for hyperintense and two for hypointense lesions), and the σ's for the Gaussian blurring. Whereas our initial idea was to train the method to find optimal parameters that would work for all images, this appeared to be unfeasible because of the variety in images and image characteristics. Therefore, in the end, we opted for a manual setting of these values per image.

3   Experiments

We used the method to de-enhance liver CECT images to assess the registration accuracy of a publicly available method for registration of diagnostic to interventional liver images. Below we describe the data, implementation and the experimental results.

3.1   Data

We retrospectively retrieved from the Erasmus MC PACS diagnostic and interventional CECT images for 20 subjects that had undergone ablation therapy for liver tumors. All imaging data was anonymized prior to processing. The Institutional Review Board (IRB) of Erasmus MC approved that the Medical Research Involving Human Subjects Act does not apply to this study and that no informed consent was required according to the local directives for retrospective studies (MEC-2014-385).

The 20 image pairs contain a total of 33 lesions, ranging from one to five lesions per patient. There were 14 patients (28 lesions) with HCCs, 6 (7) with colorectal metastases. Mean of maximum lesion diameter was 22 mm (range [11–60 mm]). CT image pixel sizes ranged from 0.6–1 mm, slice spacing ranged from 2.5–3 mm.

A trained medical student (HB) performed the manual segmentation of the liver and the lesions in both the diagnostic and interventional images using an in-house developed tool based on MeVisLab. The same person performed the de-enhancement, using an in-house developed tool build in MeVisLab. The annotation and de-enhancement was supervised by an interventional radiologist (AM) with eight years of experience.

3.2   Registration Algorithm Evaluation

We used Elastix [10] with settings according to [4] as registration algorithm. This registration algorithm uses liver masks, for which we used enlarged (dilated) versions of the manually segmented livers.

Additionally, to assess whether the presence of contrast agent in the images makes a difference for the registration, we also assessed the registration results when using the same registration approach using the original CECT images.

After registration, the resulting transformation was used to transform the lesion from the diagnostic to the interventional scan. Subsequently, the center of gravity was determined for the transformed lesion, as well as for the annotated lesion in the interventional scan. The TRE was defined as the distance between these two centers.

4   Results

4.1   De-enhancement

Table 1 lists the parameter settings statistics for the de-enhancement.

4.2   Registration Accuracy

The non-rigid registration with the VUCT images did not converge in one subject (two lesions). In these cases, the rigid registration had a very large TRE. In the other 19 subjects (31 lesions), the mean TRE for rigid registration was 10.3 mm, and for the non-rigid registration it was 5.2 mm.

The non-rigid registration with the CECT images also did not converge for one subject (same as where the VUCT registration did not converge). Over the other subjects, the mean TRE for rigid registration was 9.9 mm, and for the non-rigid registration is was 4.5 mm.

A boxplot of the errors is shown in Fig. 3, registration results are in Figs. 4 and 5.

Table 1. Parameter values for segmentation of hyper- and hypointense lesions, and parameters (α_2 and β_2) for noise distribution replacing the lesions.

Param	Hyper		Hypo	
	Mean	Stdev	Mean	Stddev
α_1	0.45	0.27	−0.092	0.57
β_1	11	5.1	−11	2.6
α_2	−0.31	0.22	0.14	0.35
β_2	0.66	0.77	1.13	0.78

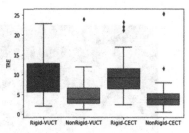

Fig. 3. TREs based on lesion centers, excluding the results of the two subjects where the non-rigid registration failed.

5 Discussion

The assessment of registration accuracy is a difficult task. In our application, the only clinically relevant metric is how well a lesion from a diagnostic image is aligned with the same lesion in the interventional image where the lesion is inconspicuous. In the past, we have used interventional unenhanced CT images for our registration development and assessment, using surrogate metrics such as Dice over the liver, liver surface distance metrics and distance between visible anatomical landmarks. The current setup allows us to assess the real TRE for our application. It is important to note that our TRE also may include errors that cannot be attributed to the registration, such as tumor growth. Whereas this metric thus not solely addressed the registration error (and thus TRE may not be the appropriate term), the error quantified is best related to the clinical practice. Additionally, the reference standard locations were the center of gravity of annotated lesions. In this way, we intended to reduce the effect of inter-observer variation and discretization errors (because of the slice spacing); small variations in annotation will have a minor effect on the center of gravity.

In a previous study involving registration of sixteen pairs of similar liver CT images [4], Luu et al. obtained a Dice overlap of 90%, a MSD of 4.6 mm and mean landmark distances of 5.3 mm. As these experiments were run on a different set of patient data (though acquired in the same hospital, with similar protocols), we should be careful in drawing strong conclusions. Still, distances are very similar to our TRE results, which suggests that the mean landmark distances are a good predictor of TRE. This may be explained by the fact that the method we used includes a term in the registration that penalizes the second derivatives of the deformation field, and thus enforces smooth deformation fields. It would be interesting to assess whether this similarity holds for other registration methods as well. The fact that the surface distance is less can be explained by the fact that this metric only takes the error orthogonal to the surface into account.

When comparing the registration results of the original CECT with the VUCT, the mean TRE of the CECT images is slightly smaller, for the rigid as well as the non-rigid registration. These differences, however, are not statisti-

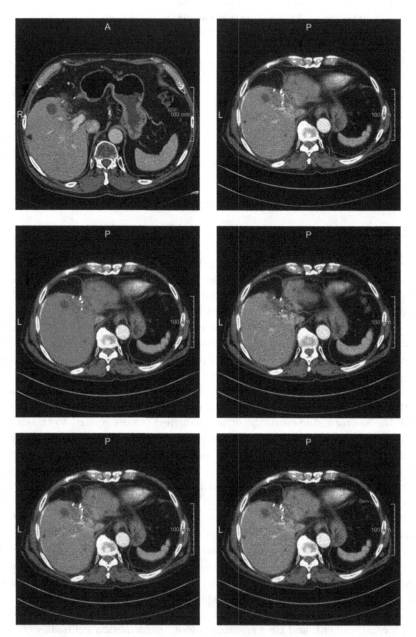

Fig. 4. Example registration result: top left: diagnostic contrast-enhanced image with annotated lesion; top right: interventional contrast-enhanced image with annotated lesion; middle left: de-enhanced image; middle right: rigid registration result (VUCT, one slice off); bottom left: VUCT registration result (lesion superimposed on VUCT image); bottom right: CECT registration result.

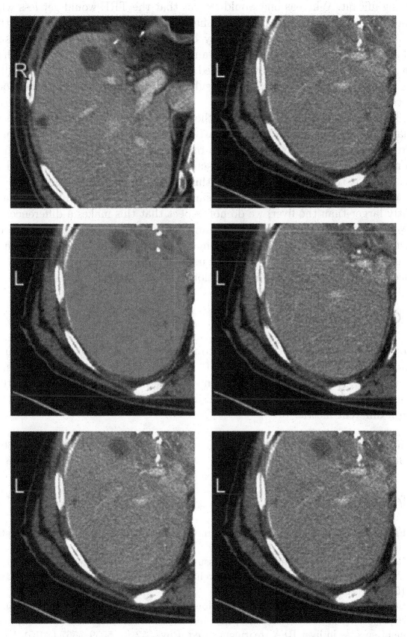

Fig. 5. Example registration result: subimages of the images in Fig. 4: top left: diagnostic contrast-enhanced image with annotated lesion; top right: interventional contrast-enhanced image with annotated lesion; middle left: de-enhanced image; middle right: rigid registration result (VUCT, one slice off); bottom left: VUCT registration result (lesion superimposed on VUCT image); bottom right: CECT registration result.

cally significant. Whereas one would expect that the TRE would get less when registering intra-model (two contrast-enhanced scans), these differences are thus not very large. One of the reasons may be that the method parameters (such as the spacing of the deformation field and the non-rigidity penalty term) have been trained with non-contrast-enhanced cases as well, and thus slightly difference settings (e.g. less penalty) may result in better results for the intra-modal registration.

The main limitation of the study is the de-enhancement process. Whereas for human observers the effect of the contrast enhancement was not visible anymore, there is no guarantee that there are no remaining effects that could be utilized by a registration approach. Also, the de-enhancement was performed on the liver only, which is the organ of interest in this study. As our registration approach used masks to limit the area where the simulation metric is computed to an area slightly larger than the liver, we do not expect that this makes a difference.

Nowadays, with dual-energy CT scanners, it is in principle possible to reconstruct a non-enhanced and a CECT image from the same contrast-enhanced acquisition. In the future, we intend to use such an approach to generate a reference standard for registration evaluation.

6   Conclusion

In conclusion, we presented a method to remove the effect of contrast enhancement for CECT images. These VUCT images were used to assess registration accuracy, focusing on the lesion centers. The non-rigid registration method applied has an error of 5.2 mm, which is similar to the results of a previous study using a different metric.

Acknowledgements. Theo van Walsum was supported by ITEA project 13031: Benefit.

References

1. Fischer, B., Modersitzki, J.: Ill-posed medicine-an introduction to image registration. Inverse Prob. **24**, 034008 (2008)
2. Rohlfing, T.: Image similarity and tissue overlaps as surrogates for image registration accuracy: widely used but unreliable. IEEE Trans. Med. Imaging. **31**(2), 153–163 (2012)
3. Luu, H.M., Klink, C., Niessen, W., Moelker, A., van Walsum, T.: An automatic registration method for pre- and post-interventional CT images for assessing treatment success in liver RFA treatment. Med. Phys. **42**(9), 5559–5567 (2015)
4. Luu, H.M., Klink, C., Niessen, W., Moelker, A., Walsum, T.V.: Non-rigid registration of liver CT images for CT-guided ablation of liver tumors. PLOS ONE **11**(9), e0161600 (2016)
5. Laura, C., Drechsler, K., Wesarg, S., Bale, R.: Accurate physics-based registration for the outcome validation of minimal invasive interventions and open liver surgeries. IEEE Trans. Biomed. Eng. **PP**(99), 1 (2016)

6. Rieder, C., Wirtz, S., Strehlow, J., Zidowitz, S., Bruners, P., Isfort, P., Mahnken, A.H., Peitgen, H.O.: Automatic alignment of pre- and post-interventional liver CT images for assessment of radiofrequency ablation, vol. 8316, pp. 83163E–83163E-8 (2012)
7. Wang, B., Ying, C.A.O.: Liver medical image registration based on biomechanical model. Multimed. Tools Appl. **76**, 1–18 (2016)
8. Nielsen, M.S., Østergaard, L.R., Carl, J.: A new method to validate thoracic CT-CT deformable image registration using auto-segmented 3D anatomical landmarks. Acta Oncol. **54**(9), 1515–1520 (2015)
9. Nie, K., Chuang, C., Kirby, N., Braunstein, S., Pouliot, J.: Site-specific deformable imaging registration algorithm selection using patient-based simulated deformations. Med. Phys. **40**(4), 041911 (2013)
10. Klein, S., Staring, M., Murphy, K., Viergever, M., Pluim, J.P.W.: Elastix: a toolbox for intensity-based medical image registration. IEEE Trans. Med. Imaging **29**(1), 196–205 (2010)

Evaluation of Multi-metric Registration for Online Adaptive Proton Therapy of Prostate Cancer

Mohamed S. Elmahdy[1](✉), Thyrza Jagt[3], Sahar Yousefi[1], Hessam Sokooti[1], Roel Zinkstok[1], Mischa Hoogeman[3], and Marius Staring[1,2]

[1] Leiden University Medical Center, Leiden, The Netherlands
m.s.e.elmahdy@lumc.nl
[2] Delft University of Technology, Delft, The Netherlands
[3] Erasmus MC Cancer Institute, Rotterdam, The Netherlands

Abstract. Delineation of the target volume and Organs-At-Risk (OARs) is a crucial step for proton therapy dose planning of prostate cancer. Adaptive proton therapy mandates automatic delineation, as manual delineation is too time consuming while it should be fast and robust. In this study, we propose an accurate and robust automatic propagation of the delineations from the planning CT to the daily CT by means of Deformable Image Registration (DIR). The proposed algorithm is a multi-metric DIR method that jointly optimizes the registration of the bladder contours and CT images. A 3D Dilated Convolutional Neural Network (DCNN) was trained for automatic bladder segmentation of the daily CT. The network was trained and tested on prostate data of 18 patients, each having 7 to 10 daily CT scans. The network achieved a Dice Similarity Coefficient (DSC) of 92.7% ± 1.6% for automatic bladder segmentation. For the automatic contour propagation of the prostate, lymph nodes, and seminal vesicles, the system achieved a DSC of 0.87 ± 0.03, 0.89 ± 0.02, and 0.67 ± 0.11 and Mean Surface Distance of 1.4 ± 0.30 mm, 1.4 ± 0.29 mm, and 1.5 ± 0.37 mm, respectively. The proposed algorithm is therefore very promising for clinical implementation in the context of online adaptive proton therapy of prostate cancer.

Keywords: Deformable image registration
Convolutional neural networks (CNN) · Prostate cancer
Proton therapy

1 Introduction

Prostate cancer is one of the leading causes of mortality and the most common cancer among men. The American Cancer Society estimates around 161,360 new cases and 26,730 deaths from prostate cancer in the United States for 2017 [1]. Intensity-Modulated Proton Therapy (IMPT) has shown the capability of delivering a highly localized dose distributions to the target volume. IMPT is

S. Klein et al. (Eds.): WBIR 2018, LNCS 10883, pp. 94–104, 2018.
https://doi.org/10.1007/978-3-319-92258-4_9

however more sensitive to daily variations that may result in a suboptimal dose distribution [2,3]. These variations could be due to anatomical changes in the target volume and Organs-At-Risk (OARs) or a misalignment in the patient positioning. In order to account for these variations, a margin is added to the Clinical Target Volume (CTV) that leads to the Planning Target Volume (PTV). These margins result in extra dose to the OARs, leading to an increase in the treatment-related toxicities that may prevent dose escalation. Repeat imaging and re-planning can handle this problem [4]. These repeat (inter-fraction) CT scans have to be delineated first before generating a new treatment plan. Therefore traditionally the inter-fraction re-contouring is not performed because it is very time consuming and consequently new anatomical changes could be introduced in the meantime. Therefore, it is vital for the automatic contouring to be fast and robust, because otherwise there will be a need for fallback strategies like manual correction that also take time.

The Atlas Based Auto Segmentation (ABAS) tool, Mirada, RayStation, and MIM softwares are a well known commercial softwares for automatic re-contouring. However, these softwares are considered a black box for the users, and therefore limits the potential of parameter customization and tuning. Open source DIR packages provide a high level of flexibility with a concrete scientific evidence and reproducibility [5,6]. Qiao et al. [7] reported an MSD of 1.36 ± 0.30 mm, 1.75 ± 0.84 mm, 1.49 ± 0.44 mm for the prostate, seminal vesicles, and lymph nodes, respectively for 18 patients using the open source elastix software. A clinical success rate of 69% was achieved, which means that 31% of the delineations have to be corrected, leading to increased costs and a suboptimal patient workflow. In 2011, Thor et al. deployed DIR to propagate the contours of the prostate and OARs from CT to cone-beam CT [8]. The system achieved a mean DSC of 0.80 for prostate, 0.77 for rectum, and 0.73 for the bladder with a relatively high variance. Moreover, the system was not qualitatively evaluated in terms of the dosimetric coverage. Recently, Woerner et al. [9] investigated the error between different radiologists and both DIR and rigid registration in different body regions. They only reported the results for the prostate, which were 0.90, 0.99 mm, and 8.12 mm for the DSC, MSD, and Hausdorff Distance (HD), respectively.

In order to improve the success rate of the automatic propagation of contours using DIR, we propose a multi-metric based registration. Hereby, instead of depending on the intensity of the images alone, we introduce a second objective that specifically optimizes the bladder overlap, based on a bladder estimate provided by a neural network.

2   Materials and Methods

2.1   Dataset

This study includes eighteen anonymized patients who were treated for prostate cancer in 2007 using intensity-modulated radiation therapy at Haukeland University Hospital. Each patient has a planning CT and 7 to 10 repeat CT scans.

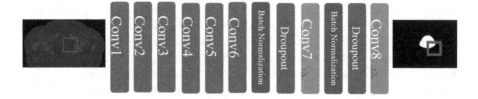

Fig. 1. The architecture for the 3D-DCNN network where $\{1X, \ldots, 16X\}$ denotes the dilation rate. The blue convolution blocks represent $3 \times 3 \times 3$ kernels while the grey convolution blocks represent fully connected convolution layers implemented by $1 \times 1 \times 1$ kernels. The green and red blocks denote batch normalization layers and dropout layers, respectively. The red square represents the patch, while the yellow square represents the receptive field. (Color figure online)

The field of view of the scans included the prostate, lymph nodes, seminal vesicles, in addition to the bladder and rectum as the main OARs. Each scan has 90 to 180 slices with a slice thickness of around 2 mm. All the slices were of size 512×512 with in-plane resolution of around 0.9 mm. The prostate, lymph nodes, seminal vesicles, rectum, and bladder were delineated in each CT scan by an expert and reviewed by another one.

2.2 Dilated Convolution Neural Network Architecture (DCNN)

Motion and filling of the bladder as well as the rectum have an important influence on the anatomical changes in the abdomen. Therefore, we hypothesize that intensity-based DIR may improve in terms of accuracy and robustness if the motion of either of these structures is taken into account explicitly. Since the bladder is a well-defined structure that is relatively easy to delineate, we opt to segment it fully automatically. In this study, we propose a 3D Dilated Convolutional Neural Network (3D-DCNN) in order to automatically segment the bladder. Dilated convolution is a generalized version of the traditional convolution process where more spacing is added to the convolution kernel so that a larger spatial neighborhood is considered when calculating the feature maps. This spacing is called the dilation rate; for traditional convolution the dilation rate is 1. Using a dilation rate larger than 1 has several advantages. First, stacking convolution layers with increasing dilation rate will accordingly enlarge the Receptive Field (RF) of the neural network without adding additional trainable parameters. Second, there is no need for adding down-sampling layers to have a large RF and therefore the network can handle high resolution volumes using a smaller number of trainable parameters. Figure 1 shows the architecture of the dilated network. This network is a modified version of the architecture deployed in [10]. The first six convolutional layers have a kernel size of $3 \times 3 \times 3$, 32 feature maps, and a logarithmic increasing dilation rate. Dropout layers with a dropout rate of 0.6 as well as batch normalization layers are introduced before the last two fully convolutional layers. Moreover, the 2D convolution layers in

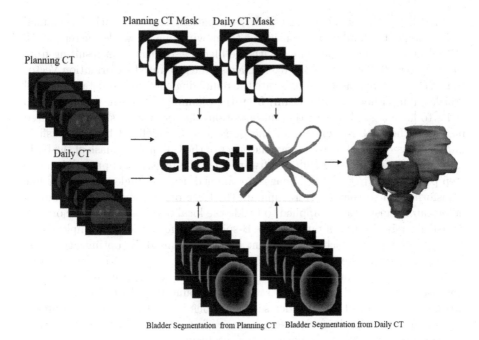

Fig. 2. The proposed multi-metric registration process using `elastix` software.

the original architecture were replaced with 3D layers in order to consider the homogeneity of tissues in 3D. Hence, it can help to get more accurate and robust results. The network has a receptive field of $65 \times 65 \times 65$ and has 144,551 trainable parameters.

In order to train the network, the 18 patients are divided into three sets: 12 patients for training, 3 patients for validation, and 3 patients for testing. This results in a total of 120, 28, and 30 CT scans for training, validation, and testing, respectively. 1,000,000 patches of size $71 \times 71 \times 71$ are randomly extracted from the training volumes, making sure they are equally distributed between foreground and background. Cross Entropy is deployed as a cost function and the network is trained using the Adam optimizer with a fixed learning rate of 10^{-4}. All the experiments were carried out using an NVIDIA GTX1080 Ti with 11 GB of GPU memory.

2.3 Image Registration

The open source package `elastix` was used for deformable image registration [6]. This package is available from http://elastix.isi.uu.nl. All the experiments were performed on a desktop PC operated on Windows 10 with 16 GB of memory and an Intel Xeon E51620 CPU with 4 cores running at 3.6 GHz.

In this study, the planning CT of each patient together with the manual delineation of the bladder are considered the moving images, while the repeat CT of the same patient accompanied with the bladder segmentation resulting from the proposed 3D-DCNN are the fixed images. The generated Deformation Vector Field (DVF) is then used to propagate the remaining contours (prostate, seminal vesicles, lymph nodes, and rectum) from the planning CT to the repeat CT. In order to have a good registration initialization, the registrations were initialized based on the center-of-gravity of the bony anatomy defined by a Hounsfield number larger than 200. To remove the effect of the CT table, a mask of the body torso was generated using Pulmo software [11]. The registration process is a two step procedure. First, the CT images are aligned using a single resolution affine transformation so that we can eliminate the large organ movements. Second, a deformable registration is applied to tackle the local deformations of the organs. A fast recursive implementation of the B-spline transformation was employed for DIR [12]. Adaptive stochastic gradient descent was used for optimization [13]. Figure 2 illustrates the proposed registration pipeline. For the DIR stage we used a three level Gaussian pyramid, and two cost functions. Mutual information was used for the CT images. To take into account the bladder contours the distance transform of the bladder segmentations is used instead of the binary segmentations themselves, to ensure a smooth and stable optimization process. This results in the following optimization problem:

$$\hat{\mu} = \arg\min_{\mu}\{C_1\left(I_F, I_M; T_\mu\right) + \alpha C_2\left(DT\left(S_F\right), DT\left(S_M\right); T_\mu\right)\}, \qquad (1)$$

where C_1 is the mutual information cost function, C_2 is the Mean Square Difference (MSD) cost function, α is a weight balancing these two cost functions, I_F is the daily scan, I_M is the planning scan, $DT\left(S_F\right)$ is the distance transform of the DCNN bladder segmentation, and $DT\left(S_M\right)$ is the distance transform of the manual annotation of the planning scan.

2.4   Registration Performance Evaluation

The registration quality is measured by the overlap and residual distance between the manually and the automatically propagated contours of the daily CT for the prostate, lymph nodes, seminal vesicles, rectum, and bladder. The most common metrics for quality are the Dice Similarity Coefficient (DSC), the Mean Surface Distance (MSD), and the Hausdorff Distance (HD), all computed in 3D.

$$DSC = \sum \frac{2|F \cap M|}{|F| + |M|}, \qquad (2)$$

where F and M are the propagated contour and the ground truth contour, respectively.

$$MSD = \frac{1}{2}\left(\frac{1}{n}\sum_{i=1}^{n} d\left(a_i, M\right) + \frac{1}{m}\sum_{i=1}^{m} d\left(b_i, F\right)\right), \qquad (3)$$

$$HD = \max \left\{ \max_i \{d\left(a_i, M\right)\}, \max_j \{d\left(b_i, F\right)\} \right\}, \tag{4}$$

where $\{a_1, a_2, ..., a_n\}$ and $\{b_1, b_2, ..., b_m\}$ are the surface mesh points of the fixed and moving contours, respectively and $d\left(a_i, M\right) = \min_j \|b_j - a_i\|$.

3   Experimental Results

3.1   DCNN Segmentation Performance

The DCNN network achieved an average segmentation DSC of 92.7% ± 1.6% on the test patients. It took an average of 15 s to segment a single volume using a single GPU depending on the number of slices per volume.

3.2   Registration Performance

The weight α of the cost function for the bladder segmentation (C_2) was set to 0.05 for the first resolution and zero for the second and third resolutions. These weights were chosen after a set of initial experiments. For investigating the effect of the number of iterations on the registration performance, we varied this parameter between 100 and 500 iterations. Table 1 illustrates the DSC evaluations of the single-metric and multi-metric registrations for the set of iterations. The overlap performance of the prostate, lymph nodes, and rectum were very similar for single and multi metric registrations. For the seminal vesicles and bladder the overlap was higher for multi-metric at 100 and 500 iterations.

The evaluations in terms of MSD are shown in Table 2. For the prostate, seminal vesicles, rectum, and bladder, there was a significant improvement from the affine transformation to DIR-100, and a slight improvement for 500 iterations in both single and multi-metric registrations. This was not the case for lymph nodes. However, the MSD errors for almost all the organs were within a voxel size. The 95% HD showed a similar pattern as MSD as presented in Table 3.

Figure 3 shows the comparison of the registration performance between single-metric (intensity image only) and multi-metric registrations (intensity and bladder segmentation) for affine, 100, and 500 iterations. The comparison illustrates the performance in terms of DSC, MSD, and 95%HD for the target volumes and OARs. The figure shows much less outliers for the multi-metric registrations, especially for the seminal vesicles, which is a challenging structure due to its small volume. Here, results above the top whisker (defined by 1.5 times the inter-quartile range) are termed an outlier. In order to explore the upper limit of the proposed method, it was tested with the manual annotation of the bladder instead of the segmentation of the DCNN. The boxplot shows a very similar pattern between the multi-metric registration using the bladder contours from the DCNN network and the manually annotated bladder contours.

Table 1. DSC value of the target volumes and OARs for different registration settings. † and ‡ represent a significant difference (at $p = 0.05$) between single-metric and multi-metric for 100 and 500 iterations, respectively.

Evaluation	# it.	Prostate	SV[†]	LN	Rectum	Bladder[†‡]
		$\mu \pm \sigma$	$\mu \pm \sigma$	$\mu \pm \sigma$	$\mu \pm \sigma$	$\mu \pm \sigma$
Affine		0.83 ± 0.08	0.34 ± 0.27	0.92 ± 0.03	0.69 ± 0.09	0.78 ± 0.07
Single-metric	100	0.87 ± 0.03	0.59 ± 0.22	0.90 ± 0.02	0.77 ± 0.08	0.90 ± 0.05
	500	0.87 ± 0.04	0.63 ± 0.20	0.89 ± 0.02	0.78 ± 0.07	0.91 ± 0.06
Multi-metric	100	0.87 ± 0.03	0.67 ± 0.11	0.89 ± 0.02	0.78 ± 0.06	0.93 ± 0.03
	500	0.87 ± 0.02	0.66 ± 0.11	0.89 ± 0.02	0.79 ± 0.06	0.93 ± 0.03

Table 2. MSD (mm) of the target volumes and OARs for different registration settings. † and ‡ represent a significant difference (at $p = 0.05$) between single-metric and multi-metric for 100 and 500 iterations, respectively.

Evaluation	# it.	Prostate	SV[†]	LN	Rectum	Bladder[†‡]
		$\mu \pm \sigma$	$\mu \pm \sigma$	$\mu \pm \sigma$	$\mu \pm \sigma$	$\mu \pm \sigma$
Affine		1.8 ± 0.78	3.7 ± 2.00	1.1 ± 0.37	4.1 ± 1.50	4.3 ± 1.70
Single-metric	100	1.4 ± 0.33	2.1 ± 1.40	1.3 ± 0.28	3.1 ± 1.30	2.0 ± 1.00
	500	1.3 ± 0.35	1.9 ± 1.40	1.4 ± 0.27	3.0 ± 1.20	1.7 ± 0.87
Multi-metric	100	1.4 ± 0.30	1.5 ± 0.37	1.4 ± 0.29	2.9 ± 0.95	1.4 ± 0.38
	500	1.3 ± 0.28	1.6 ± 0.42	1.4 ± 0.29	2.8 ± 0.88	1.3 ± 0.32

Table 3. %95HD (mm) of the target volumes and OARs for different registration settings. † and ‡ represent a significant difference (at $p = 0.05$) between single-metric and multi-metric for 100 and 500 iterations, respectively.

Evaluation	# it.	Prostate	SV[†‡]	LN	Rectum	Bladder[†‡]
		$\mu \pm \sigma$	$\mu \pm \sigma$	$\mu \pm \sigma$	$\mu \pm \sigma$	$\mu \pm \sigma$
Affine		4.0 ± 1.70	7.8 ± 3.7	2.7 ± 1.00	11.0 ± 4.7	11.0 ± 4.7
Single-metric	100	3.2 ± 0.96	5.2 ± 3.3	3.3 ± 0.63	9.5 ± 4.3	5.9 ± 3.9
	500	3.1 ± 1.00	4.9 ± 3.4	3.4 ± 0.63	9.3 ± 4.2	5.0 ± 3.4
Multi-metric	100	3.2 ± 0.97	4.0 ± 1.5	3.6 ± 0.71	8.7 ± 3.4	3.4 ± 1.4
	500	3.0 ± 1.00	4.1 ± 1.5	3.6 ± 0.71	8.5 ± 3.2	3.2 ± 1.1

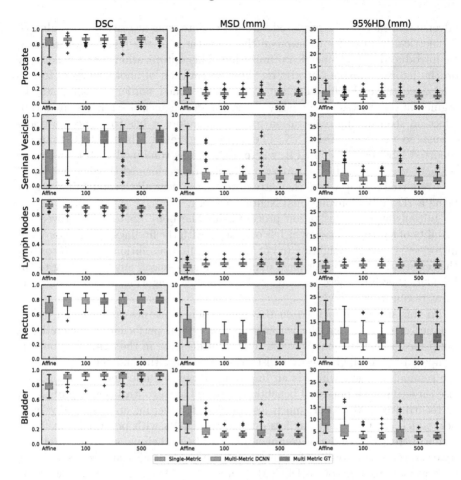

Fig. 3. Boxplot comparison between single-metric and multi-metric image registration versus the number of iterations. The columns show the DSC, MSD, and 95%HD from left to right. Prostate, seminal vesicles, lymph nodes, rectum, and bladder are shown from top to bottom rows, respectively. Here multi-metric DCNN is the result of using the bladder segmentation of the network, while multi-metric GT is the result of using the ground truth bladder delineation.

4 Discussion and Conclusion

In this study, we investigated the hypothesis of enhancing the performance and robustness of the automatic contouring of the target volumes and OARs for prostate cancer using multi-metric Deformable Image Registration (DIR). The purpose of adaptive IMPT is to be able to use a small margin between PTV and CTV, which is only a viable option if the daily re-planning can be performed in an accurate and robust manner. This daily re-planning requires robust automatic re-contouring in order to avoid local treatment-related toxicities and subsequent adverse side effects. The proposed automatic contouring algorithm was evaluated geometrically. In order to improve the robustness of the registration process, we introduced a multi-metric optimization. This optimization depends not only on the intensity image but also on the segmentation of another organ. In this study, we chose the bladder due to its well defined borders which eases the segmentation process. The quality of the bladder segmentation has a significant effect on steering the registration process, therefore it has to be accurate and robust, so we chose 3D-DCNN. The network achieved a higher DSC than the reported DSC of 81.9% in [14], where a CNN was combined with level sets to segment the bladder in CT urography. It also outperformed the dice overlap of 72% reported in [15], where they attempted to segment all the abdominal organs using a 2D Fully Convolutional Neural Network.

Initializing the registration process using the bony anatomy improved the stability of the registration which is consistent with the findings in [13]. Moreover, introducing a small weighting (α) of 0.05 at the first resolution managed to steer the registration to a better local minima without causing any overfitting to the bladder, therefore there was no need for further weighting in the second and third resolutions.

In this study, we focused on the registration robustness represented by the number of outliers and the variance in the system performance. Overall, the multi-metric registration showed a significant decrease in the number of outliers compared to the single-metric registration. Reducing the number of outliers for the seminal vesicles, which is an important target volume, means a more precise targeting with potential benefits in terms of local control (lower probability of recurrences). Moreover, much less outliers for rectum and especially bladder, which are OARs, means less dose to the OARs with potential benefits in terms of treatment-induced complications after the therapy, so higher probability of better quality-of-life after treatment, see Fig. 3. It also showed a significant improvement in terms of the DSC, MSD, and 95% HD for the seminal vesicles and bladder. For multi-metric registration, the overall performance gets slightly better for 500 iterations and remarkably increased from affine transformation. The figure shows a similar pattern between the multi-metric registration using the manually annotated contours of the bladder and the contours from the DCNN network. This pattern emphasizes that, the proposed method achieved the upper limit of the system. For most of the organs, the registration performance in terms of the MSD was less than 2 mm, which is less than the slice thickness.

In this study, we illustrated the effectiveness of deploying multi-metric registration using the elastix software in order to automatically re-contour daily CT scans of the prostate. This re-contouring showed a promise for generating daily treatment plans. Moreover, it showed a substantial improvement in the system robustness, which means that more treatment plans can be directly used without manual correction, which is a crucial factor for enabling online daily adaptation and thus the use of relatively small treatment margins. Therefore, the proposed method could facilitate online adaptive proton therapy of prostate cancer.

Acknowledgments. This study was financially supported by ZonMw, the Netherlands Organization for Health Research and Development, grant number 104003012. The CT-data with contours were collected at Haukeland University Hospital, Bergen, Norway and were provided to us by responsible oncologist Svein Inge Helle and physicist Liv Bolstad Hysing; they are gratefully acknowledged.

References

1. American Cancer Society. https://www.cancer.org/cancer/prostate-cancer/about/key-statistics.html
2. Zhang, M., Westerly, D., Mackie, T.: Introducing an on-line adaptive procedure for prostate image guided intensity modulate proton therapy. Phys. Med. Biol. **56**(15), 4947–4965 (2011)
3. Lomax, A.: Intensity modulated proton therapy and its sensitivity to treatment uncertainties 1: the potential effects of calculational uncertainties. Phys. Med. Biol. **53**(4), 1027–1042 (2008)
4. Hansen, E., Bucci, M., Quivey, J., Weinberg, V., Xia, P.: Repeat CT imaging and replanning during the course of IMRT for head-and-neck cancer. Int. J. Radiat. Oncol. Biol. Phys. **64**(2), 355–362 (2006)
5. Yang, D., Brame, S., El Naqa, I., Aditya, A., Wu, Y., Murty Goddu, S., Mutic, S., Deasy, J., Low, D.: Technical note: DIRART- a software suite for deformable image registration and adaptive radiotherapy research. Med. Phys. **38**(1), 67–77 (2010)
6. Klein, S., Staring, M., Murphy, K., Viergever, M., Pluim, J.: elastix: a toolbox for intensity-based medical image registration. IEEE Trans. Med. Imaging **29**(1), 196–205 (2010)
7. Qiao, Y.: Fast optimization methods for image registration in adaptive radiation therapy. Ph.D. thesis, Leiden University Medical Center (2017)
8. Thor, M., Petersen, J., Bentzen, L., HØyer, M., Muren, L.: Deformable image registration for contour propagation from CT to cone-beam CT scans in radiotherapy of prostate cancer. Acta Oncologica **50**(6), 918–925 (2011)
9. Woerner, A., Choi, M., Harkenrider, M., Roeske, J., Surucu, M.: Evaluation of deformable image registration-based contour propagation from planning CT to cone-beam CT. Technol. Cancer Res. Treat. **16**(6), 801–810 (2017)
10. Wolterink, J.M., Leiner, T., Viergever, M.A., Išgum, I.: Dilated convolutional neural networks for cardiovascular MR segmentation in congenital heart disease. In: Zuluaga, M.A., Bhatia, K., Kainz, B., Moghari, M.H., Pace, D.F. (eds.) RAMBO/HVSMR -2016. LNCS, vol. 10129, pp. 95–102. Springer, Cham (2017). https://doi.org/10.1007/978-3-319-52280-7_9
11. Staring, M., Bakker, M., Stolk, J., Shamonin, D., Reiber, J., Stoel, B.: Towards local progression estimation of pulmonary emphysema using CT. Med. Phys. **41**(2), 021905 (2014)
12. Huizinga, W., Klein, S., Poot, D.H.J.: Fast multidimensional B-spline interpolation using template metaprogramming. In: Ourselin, S., Modat, M. (eds.) WBIR 2014. LNCS, vol. 8545, pp. 11–20. Springer, Cham (2014). https://doi.org/10.1007/978-3-319-08554-8_2
13. Qiao, Y., van Lew, B., Lelieveldt, B.P.F., Staring, M.: Fast automatic step size estimation for gradient descent optimization of image registration. IEEE Trans. Med. Imaging **35**(2), 391–403 (2016)

14. Cha, K.H., Hadjiiski, L., Samala, R.K., Chan, H.-P., Caoili, E.M., Cohan, R.H.: Urinary bladder segmentation in CT urography using deep-learning convolutional neural network and level sets. Med. Phys. **43**(4), 1882–1896 (2016)

15. Zhou, X., Ito, T., Takayama, R., Wang, S., Hara, T., Fujita, H.: Three-dimensional CT image segmentation by combining 2D fully convolutional network with 3D majority voting. In: Carneiro, G., et al. (eds.) LABELS/DLMIA -2016. LNCS, vol. 10008, pp. 111–120. Springer, Cham (2016). https://doi.org/10.1007/978-3-319-46976-8_12

Instrument Pose Estimation Using Registration for Otobasis Surgery

David Kügler[✉], Martin Andrade Jastrzebski, and Anirban Mukhopadhyay

Department for Computer Science, TU Darmstadt, Darmstadt, Germany
{david.kuegler,anirban.mukhopadhyay}@gris.tu-darmstadt.de

Abstract. Clinical outcome of several Minimally Invasive Surgeries (MIS) heavily depend on the accuracy of intraoperative pose estimation of the surgical instrument from intraoperative x-rays. The estimation consists of finding the tool in a given set of x-rays and extracting the necessary data to recreate the tool's pose for further navigation - resulting in severe consequences of incorrect estimation. Though state-of-the-art MIS literature has exploited image registration as a tool for instrument pose estimation, lack of practical considerations in previous study design render their conclusion ineffective from a clinical standpoint. One major issue of such a study is the lack of Ground Truth in clinical data -as there are no direct ways of measuring the ground truth pose and indirect estimation accumulates error. A systematic way to overcome this problem is to generate Digitally Reconstructed Radiographs (DRR), however, such procedure generates data which are free from measuring errors (e.g. noise, number of projections), resulting claims of registration performance inconclusive. Generalization of registration performance across different instruments with different Degrees of Freedom (DoF) has not been studied as well. By marrying a rigorous study design involving several clinical scenarios with, for example, several optimizers, metrics and others parameters for image registration, this paper bridges this gap effectively. Although the pose estimation error scales inversely with instrument size, we show image registration generalizes well for different instruments and DoF. In particular, it is shown that increasing the number of x-ray projections can reduce the pose estimation error significantly across instruments - which might lead to the acquisition of several x-rays for pose estimation in a clinical workflow.

1 Introduction

Minimally Invasive Surgeries (MIS) presents several advantages over conventional open surgical procedures since they require smaller incisions, resulting in reduced trauma and lowered risk of infection [1,2]. As a result, MIS is becoming increasingly popular across several surgical disciplines where traditionally an open procedure with higher clinical risk was the only option e.g. bone surgery [3]. However, the ability of avoiding risk structures for such MIS procedures is limited by the accuracy of the estimation of the surgical instrument's pose from

© Springer International Publishing AG, part of Springer Nature 2018
S. Klein et al. (Eds.): WBIR 2018, LNCS 10883, pp. 105–114, 2018.
https://doi.org/10.1007/978-3-319-92258-4_10

intraoperative x-ray. Consequently instrument pose estimation has direct impact to the clinical outcome of MIS. Major challenges to overcome for this pose estimation task are the obstruction of line-of-sight, the reduced size of the tools, and the lack of haptic feedback [4].

We consider MIS at the otobasis, where multiple clinical tasks require drilling, e.g. cochlear implant, tumor resection, specific point drug delivery and several other procedures. The feasibility and success of these interventions rely heavily on precise navigation, which is currently ensured by removing the bone to provide line-of-sight. Reliable and accurate pose estimation of the surgical instrument is therefore a prerequisite of MIS in this region. In this paper, we study the generalization ability of image registration techniques for pose estimation of several instruments from intraoperative x-ray images during MIS at otobasis.

Several aspects of image registration have been studied for instrument pose estimation in a general MIS [5–7] setting. For example, Rivaz et al. [8] studied several image comparison metrics in different pose estimation setups. Similarly, influence of image features on registration have been studied as well [9]. Additionally impact of optimizers and regularizers on the registration quality has been studied. For example, Kelner et al. [10], proposed a hybrid optimization technique to overcome limitations inherent to specific metrics, methods and setups. On the other hand, Peng et al. [11] and Russakoff et al. [12] explored novel methods to execute the registration. Kügler et al. [13] even replaced Metric and Opimizer by a convolutional neural network. Williamson et al. [3] studied ways to estimate the pose of a robot-guided surgical drill tool based on the correlation of the drilling force and the bone density in the mastoid extracted from 3-D image data and was able to estimate it with a mean accuracy of 0.29 mm.

While those works present a variety of registration approaches for instrument pose estimation, one crucial element of such study design namely valid ground truth has not been studied properly. This is a major challenge for the evaluation of pose estimation techniques. Most of those studies use Fiducial Markers on phantoms for reference measurement. But this leaves us with no control over the conditions of the images such as noise. In addition to that, the instrument's pose can only be described if the projection parameters of the c-arm machine are known and this requires a large volume of data, such as the positions of the instrument, the detector and the source. The expected accuracy required for a valid evaluation of the pose estimation becomes a challenge due to the projection nature of the c-arm.

To circumvent this problem, we opted to use Digitally Rendered Radiographs (DRRs) as fixed images to have a ground truth reference position. However, unlike simpler studies where DRRs generate noise free acquisitions, artificial noise was added to our generated images simulating known problems inherent to image acquisition due to electronic noise [14]. This resulted in simulated x-rays very similar in appearance to he ones acquired in practical MIS scenarios.

The Major contribution of this paper is the development of a rigorous evaluation framework to study the performance of image registration techniques during MIS at the Otobasis, which involves two different instruments with different sizes and number of Degrees of Freedom (DoFs) as well as the effects of noise, optimizers and metrics (Fig. 1).

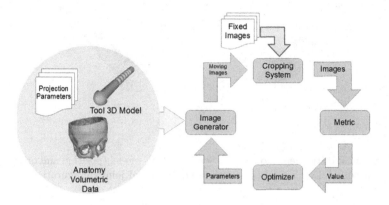

Fig. 1. ITK based registration loop

2   Methods

This paper presents a study of the use of 2D x-ray images for the estimation of surgical instrument's poses with 6 or 8 DoFs and the impact of acquisition setups on the accuracy of this estimation.

Problem Definition: Let $\mathcal{P} = (P_1, \cdots, P_n)$ be a set of projection matrices used to obtain the reference radiographs $\mathcal{S} = (I_1(P_1), \cdots, I_n(P_n))$ showing the instrument, whose pose we want to estimate.

For $\theta = (\theta_1, \cdots, \theta_k)$ describing the pose and the configuration of a model M similar to the instrument, we have a generator capable of generating a set of n DRRs $\mathcal{S}'(\theta, \mathcal{P}) = (I_1'(P_1), \cdots, I_n'(P_n))$ using the same projection matrices.

Given a similarity metric $\mathcal{F}(I, I')$ with I and I' two radiographs, we define the task of instrument pose estimation through registration as the search for the set of parameters $\hat{\theta} = (\theta_1, \cdots, \theta_k)$ which maximize the similarity A of the sets of reference $\mathcal{S}$ and generated $\mathcal{S}'$ radiographs:

$$\hat{\theta} = \arg\max_{\theta} \sum_i^n A = \arg\max_{\theta} \sum_i^n \mathcal{F}(\mathcal{S}_i, \mathcal{S}'_i(\theta)) \tag{1}$$

In this paper θ has 6 and 8 components for two different instruments leading to 6 and 8 DoFs optimization problems respectively.

In summary, the inputs to our registration method are the reference images $\mathcal{S}$, the projection parameters $\mathcal{P}$, a 3D model of the instrument (mesh) M, an initial estimate of the instruments pose $\hat{\theta}^{t=0}$ and a computer tomography volume scan of the surrounding anatomy V. The method generates sets of DRRs

$\mathcal{S}'(\hat{\theta}^t, \mathcal{P})$ and by increasing the similarity measure A between the reference and the generated radiographs, finds better estimates of the ground truth pose $\theta_{gt} = (\theta_{gt,1}, \cdots, \theta_{gt,n})$ of the instrument w.r.t. the camera.

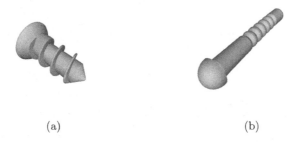

(a)   (b)

Fig. 2. Surgical instrument models: (a) Screw - 6 DoF model (position and orientation) and (b) Robot - 8 DoF model (position, orientation and joint configuration)

Implementation Concept: Our approach implements this parameter search as an optimization loop based on the Insight Registration and Segmentation Toolkit (ITK) [15] following Algorithm 1.

We apply the Correlation Coefficient (CC) and Mutual Information (MI) metrics ($\mathcal{F} = \mathcal{F}_{CC}$ or $\mathcal{F} = \mathcal{F}_{MI}$) to compare the respective fixed and moving images. Correlation Coefficient is a symmetrical measure of linear dependence between two random variables that relates to the various correlation measures that have been used in image registration.

Mutual Information, on the other hand, only assumes a high likelihood of "consistent intensity mappings". Therefore two images are similar, if in a pixel-wise comparison of image-intensities the same mappings between intensities reoccur repeatedly. MI is robust against non-linear intensity mappings by design.

While the 6 DoF screw-model's parameters include the spatial position (x, y, z) and the orientation (O_x, O_y, O_z), the 8 DoF robot-model extends these adding parameters that describe the flexing α and the extension J_{ext} of its joint. The joint of the robot spans the bellows section (Fig. 2b). The main diameter for both instruments is approx. 3 mm.

Algorithm 1. Registration Algorithm

    Input: $\mathcal{P}, \mathcal{S}, \hat{\theta}^{t=0}(\theta_1, \cdots), M, V$
    Output: $\hat{\theta}^{t_{max}}$

1 **for** t **in** $1, \cdots, t_{max}$ **do**
2     $M^t \leftarrow$ Deform Mesh $(\hat{\theta}^{t-1})$
3     $\mathcal{S}' \leftarrow$ Generate DRRs $(\hat{\theta}^{t-1}, \mathcal{P})$
4     $A \leftarrow \sum_i^n \mathcal{F}(\mathcal{S}_i, \mathcal{S}'_i)$
5     $\hat{\theta}^t \leftarrow$ Optimize (A)
6 **end**

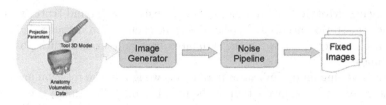

Fig. 3. Ground truth images generation.

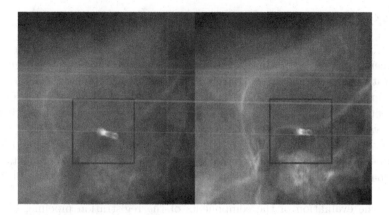

Fig. 4. Example fixed and moving image, the image part actually used for the registration is highlighted in red. (Color figure online)

Since a trustworthy ground truth is a prerequisite for any well defined evaluation of the registration quality, we generate fixed images artificially. The ground truth poses are calculated geometrically and their errors are therefore negligible.

In order to simulate differences in the acquisition of fixed and moving images we introduce a distortion pipeline to simulate common x-ray properties. This pipeline consists of an non-linear image intensity distortion and noise generators as illustrated in Fig. 3. The noise generator simulates the Gaussian noise that occurs in radiographs and is independent of tissue attenuation [14]. The non-linear distortion filter (sigmoid filter) simulates the attenuation and detector-response applying a pixel-wise transformation (Eq. 2) of the intensity to both the computer tomography volume and the projections simulating varying x-ray and detector properties:

$$f(x) = (f_{Max} - f_{Min}) * \frac{1}{1 + e^{-(x-b)/a}} + f_{Min} \tag{2}$$

f_{Max} and f_{Min} denote the maximum and minimum intensity values of the image respectively. The transformation parameters a and b define the non-linearity and the normalization of the transformation. Finally, the images are cut to regions of interest centered around the currently evaluated position of the instrument projected onto the image. Figure 4 shows a moving and a fixed image and highlights the selection of the region of interest.

Evaluation Metrics: Making use of this transformed ground truth, we evaluate the registration accuracy by the mean linear euclidean distance L_d and the angular difference A_d between the estimated pose and ground truth pose of the fixed image.

Despite being an optimization parameter, we ignore the rotation around the symmetry axis for the evaluation of the 6 DoF model. We ignore this rotation, since it is ambiguous, hard to determine and not relevant for our application.

3   Experiments

We performed 8 different experiments corresponding to Figs. 5a and 6b with multiple scenarios as deviations from the standard scenario: 35 dB of peak signal-to-noise ratio, 2 projections, the Covariance Matrix Adaptation Evolution Strategy as optimizer and Coefficient Correlation. We performed 50 registration runs for each scenario. We limited each run was limited to 400 iterations of the optimizer, which was typically enough to achieve convergence.

We seed the initial estimate of the instrument pose with the ground truth instrument pose plus a random perturbation of the individual components. The perturbation was drawn component-wise from a Uniform distribution of 2 mm and 2°.

For the evaluation of the components of the registration pipeline, we performed the tests using the 6 DoF model. We additionally evaluated the approach on the 8 DoF model to generalize the results on the deformable instrument.

As stated by Bouget et al. [16] one of the limiting factors of the fast development of technology in image registration is the lack of established surgical tool data-sets and ranking of methods. We compared the performance of Mutual Information and Coefficient Correlation (c.f. Fig. 5a).

The comparison of three different optimizers (One-plus-One, Amoeba and CMA) extends this methodological analysis (c.f. Fig. 5b).

To our knowledge no analysis of the impact of image noise has been presented with a focus on surgical instruments. We evaluated the effect of noise for both instruments using Mutual Information (Fig. 5c for the screw and Fig. 5d for the robot model respectively).

We varied the size of the 6 DoF instrument, to determine the impact of instrument size on the pose estimation task. Although the detection of small objects is a studied in computer vision as a whole, to our knowledge no analysis has not been performed in the context of surgical instruments yet.

Separating c-arm and instrument pose estimation accuracies, we evaluated how small imprecisions of the c-arm pose estimation (patient w.r.t. the c-arm) influence the instrument pose estimation. We applied a small perturbation to the ground truth Projection Parameters of 3.5° on the expected orientation of the c-arm. This value is consistent with the upper range of possible positioning calibration errors of a c-arm found by Silva et al. [17], who presented results of $1.5° \pm 1.3°$ and $1.8° \pm 1.7°$ depending on axis. We evaluated the resulting error for both models (c.f. Fig. 5f).

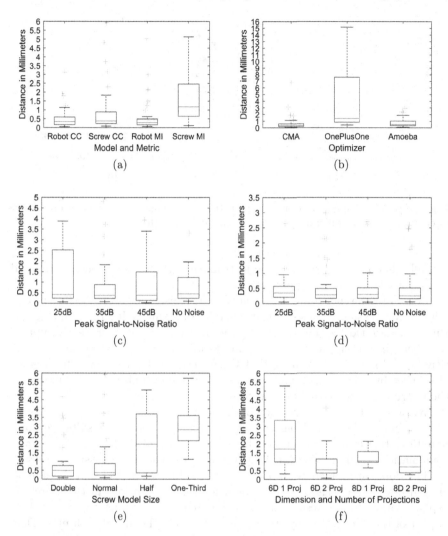

Fig. 5. Comparison of experimental scenarios: (a) Metrics, (b) Optimizers, effect of noise (for screw (c) and robot (d)), (e) Size of instrument (for screw) and (f) Projection parameters inaccuracy

Finally, we performed an analysis of the number of projections used for the registration for both models (Fig. 6a) and using different noise levels (Fig. 6b).

4 Results and Discussion

We were able to achieve average pose estimation accuracies of 0.4 mm for both models. These results are comparable to those of Otake *et al.* [18], Uneri *et al.*

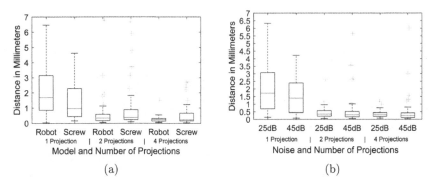

Fig. 6. Quantitative comparison to demonstrate the impact of number of projections in combination with different instruments (a) and noise (b)

[5] and others, because the surgical instruments, whose pose is being estimated, is typically larger in these publications.

Regarding the choice of components for the registration loop, Coefficient Correlation Metric showed better results than Mattes Mutual Information (Fig. 5a). But as mentioned by Markelj *et al.* [7] no method can be seen clearly superior to other, since each one can be the most suitable to be used in some specific situations. Figure 5b illustrates, that CMA performed better than the Amoeba Optimizer by a factor of 2 and the One-plus-One optimizer is not suitable for the instrument pose estimation problem.

We observed a small correlation of the accuracy to the noise level (c.f. Figs. 5c and d), but in the overall bigger picture of comparisons the results are dominated by other evaluated factors. Therefore we concluded, that the investigated combination of MI and CMA is largely robust to pixel-wise gaussian noise.

The dominating factors are the model (c.f. Figs. 5a and c) and the number of projections (see Figs. 6a and b) used for the registration. In the search for explanations, why the results are so dominated by the model, we analyzed the impact of the size of the object. We did not expect the model with more DoFs to consistently outperform the simpler model in the evaluation. Although the diameters of both models were approximately the same, the length of the models is different with the screw (6 DoF) being shorter than the robot (6 DoF). Comparing the registration accuracy of different sized screws, we observed a strong relationship between the instrument size and the pose estimation accuracy. With this dependence on the instrument size, we are confident the method generalizes to different instruments, but an initialization quality dependent on the instrument size is required.

The ambiguity of different parameters of the robot model lead to optimizations ending in local minima. We observed the following examples of local minima for the optimizer: The optimizer mistook changes in z-depth for variations of the joint extension or the limited change of the model geometry by rotation around the instruments axis was not correctly interpreted. The registration could be stabilized by using additional projections (c.f. Figs. 6a and b), leading to better pose estimation results. The largest contributions of the error in registrations using one projections can be contributed to faulty depth-estimation. Interestingly, the registration leads to better results for the image coordinate in one projection than in even in the best of multiple projections.

5 Conclusion

Surgical pose estimation by image registration estimates the pose of surgical instruments with the potential to aid doctors in understanding where instruments are located, if they cannot be seen directly. For Computer-Aided Interventions in MIS, the possibility to measure the pose of manipulated instruments using x-rays may open new opportunities and may provide options if line-of-sight is impeded.

But to effectively use registration for otobasis surgery, methods capable of greater accuracy for smaller instruments are required, for example for the estimation of the electrode in cochlear implant insertion or placement control.

We show pose estimation with image registration generalizes across different instruments and can aid surgeons and automated procedure gain better knowledge of the interaction between the instruments and the patient. In the future this could lead to image-registration-based navigation schemes being introduced for a wide range of surgical applications.

References

1. Sauer, F.: Image registration: enabling technology for image guided surgery and therapy. In: Conference Proceedings: ... Annual International Conference of the IEEE Engineering in Medicine and Biology Society. IEEE Engineering in Medicine and Biology Society. Annual Conference, vol. 7, pp. 7242–7245 (2005)
2. Vitiello, V., Lee, S.-L., Cundy, T.P., Yang, G.-Z.: Emerging robotic platforms for minimally invasive surgery. IEEE Rev. Biomed. Eng. **6**, 111–126 (2013)
3. Williamson, T.M., Bell, B.J., Gerber, N., Salas, L., Zysset, P., Caversaccio, M., Weber, S.: Estimation of tool pose based on force-density correlation during robotic drilling. IEEE Trans. Biomed. Eng. **60**(4), 969–976 (2013)
4. Tonutti, M., Elson, D.S., Yang, G.-Z., Darzi, A.W., Sodergren, M.H.: The role of technology in minimally invasive surgery: state of the art, recent developments and future directions. Postgrad. Med. J. **93**(1097), 159–167 (2017)
5. Uneri, A., de Silva, T., Goerres, J., Jacobson, M.W., Ketcha, M.D., Reaungamornrat, S., Kleinszig, G., Vogt, S., Khanna, A.J., Osgood, G.M., Wolinsky, J.-P., Siewerdsen, J.H.: Intraoperative evaluation of device placement in spine surgery using known-component 3D–2D image registration. Phys. Med. Biol. **62**(8), 3330–3351 (2017)
6. Prisacariu, V.A., Reid, I.D.: PWP3D: real-time segmentation and tracking of 3D objects. Int. J. Comput. Vision **98**(3), 335–354 (2012)
7. Markelj, P., Tomaževič, D., Likar, B., Pernuš, F.: A review of 3D/2D registration methods for image-guided interventions. Med. Image Anal. **16**(3), 642–661 (2012)

8. Rivaz, H., Karimaghaloo, Z., Collins, D.L.: Self-similarity weighted mutual information: a new nonrigid image registration metric. Med. Image Anal. **18**(2), 343–358 (2014)
9. Oksuz, I., Mukhopadhyay, A., Bevilacqua, M., Dharmakumar, R., Tsaftaris, S.A.: Dictionary learning based image descriptor for myocardial registration of CP-BOLD MR. In: Navab, N., Hornegger, J., Wells, W.M., Frangi, A.F. (eds.) MICCAI 2015. LNCS, vol. 9350, pp. 205–213. Springer, Cham (2015). https://doi.org/10.1007/978-3-319-24571-3_25
10. Kelner, V., Capitanescu, F., Léonard, O., Wehenkel, L.: A hybrid optimization technique coupling an evolutionary and a local search algorithm. J. Comput. Appl. Math. **215**(2), 448–456 (2008)
11. Peng, X., Chen, Q., Wei, B.: An efficient medical image registration method based on mutual information model. In: 2010 Seventh International Conference on Fuzzy Systems and Knowledge Discovery (FSKD), pp. 2168–2172 (2010)
12. Russakoff, D.B., Tomasi, C., Rohlfing, T., Maurer, C.R.: Image similarity using mutual information of regions. In: Pajdla, T., Matas, J. (eds.) ECCV 2004. LNCS, vol. 3023, pp. 596–607. Springer, Heidelberg (2004). https://doi.org/10.1007/978-3-540-24672-5_47
13. Kügler, D., Stefanov, A., Mukhopadhyay, A.: i3PosNet: Instrument Pose Estimation from X-Ray. arXiv preprint http://arxiv.org/pdf/1802.09575 (2018)
14. Hilts, M., Duzenli, C.: Image filtering for improved dose resolution in CT polymer gel dosimetry. Med. phys. **31**(1), 39–49 (2004)
15. Yoo, T.S., Ackerman, M.J., Lorensen, W.E., Schroeder, W., Chalana, V., Aylward, S., Metaxas, D., Whitaker, R.: Engineering and algorithm design for an image processing Api: a technical report on ITK-the Insight Toolkit. Stud. Health Technol. Inform. **85**, 586–592 (2002)
16. Bouget, D., Allan, M., Stoyanov, D., Jannin, P.: Vision-based and marker-less surgical tool detection and tracking: a review of the literature. Med. Image Anal. **35**, 633–654 (2017)
17. de Silva, T., Punnoose, J., Uneri, A., Goerres, J., Jacobson, M., Ketcha, M.D., Manbachi, A., Vogt, S., Kleinszig, G., Khanna, A.J., Wolinksy, J.-P., Osgood, G., Siewerdsen, J.H.: C-arm positioning using virtual fluoroscopy for image-guided surgery. In: Proceedings of SPIE-the International Society for Optical Engineering, p. 10135 (2017)
18. Otake, Y., Schafer, S., Stayman, J.W., Zbijewski, W., Kleinszig, G., Graumann, R., Khanna, A.J., Siewerdsen, J.H.: Automatic localization of vertebral levels in x-ray fluoroscopy using 3D–2D registration: a tool to reduce wrong-site surgery. Phys. Med. Biol. **57**(17), 5485–5508 (2012)

Local Image Registration Uncertainty Estimation Using Polynomial Chaos Expansions

Gokhan Gunay[1(✉)], Sebastian van der Voort[1], Manh Ha Luu[1],
Adriaan Moelker[2], and Stefan Klein[1]

[1] Departments of Radiology and Medical Informatics,
Biomedical Imaging Group Rotterdam, Erasmus MC, Rotterdam, The Netherlands
g.gunay@erasmusmc.nl
[2] Departments of Radiology and Nuclear Medicine, Erasmus MC,
Rotterdam, The Netherlands

Abstract. Most image registration methods involve multiple user-defined tuning parameters, such as regularization weights and smoothing parameters. Changing these tuning parameters leads to differences in the local deformation estimates that result from the registration algorithm. Uncertainty in the optimal value of the tuning parameters thus leads to uncertainty in the local deformation estimates. In this work, we propose a method to quantify this uncertainty using an efficient surrogate modeling approach based on polynomial chaos expansion. Given a specified distribution on each input tuning parameter, this approach requires only a few image registration runs to characterize the distribution of output deformation estimates at each voxel. In experiments on liver CT images, we evaluate the accuracy of the uncertainty estimate by comparing with a brute force Monte Carlo estimate. The results show that there is a negligible difference between estimates of Monte-Carlo simulation and the proposed method. The proposed method thus provides a good indication of the uncertainty in local deformation estimates due to uncertainty in the optimal setting of tuning parameters.

Keywords: Image registration · Uncertainty estimation
Polynomial chaos expansion · Surrogate modeling

1 Introduction

Image registration (IR) is an essential task in medical imaging, aimed at finding spatial relations between images [15]. Most IR methods include multiple user-defined parameters such as penalty weights and smoothing parameters. The performance of IR is heavily affected by these parameters. They need to be tuned so as to obtain desired IR outcomes and changes in these parameters cause variations in the local deformation estimates resulting from the IR algorithm. The optimal values of the tuning parameters are uncertain. This uncertainty causes

© Springer International Publishing AG, part of Springer Nature 2018
S. Klein et al. (Eds.): WBIR 2018, LNCS 10883, pp. 115–125, 2018.
https://doi.org/10.1007/978-3-319-92258-4_11

uncertainty in the local deformation estimates. Quantification and visualization of this uncertainty would be helpful in assessing the reliability of the registration results.

For a single tuning parameter, a straightforward solution to estimate IR uncertainty due to uncertainty in that tuning parameter would be to perform a Monte Carlo simulation, simply running the IR for different values of the tuning parameter sampled from its prior distribution. However, this approach would become prohibitively computationally demanding for multiple tuning parameters, as the number of required sampling points increases exponentially due to the curse of dimensionality. In the literature, several studies have focused on uncertainty estimation for IR. Kybic [7] presented a method to quantify the uncertainty due to the stochastic nature of the images, using a bootstrapping approach. Muenzing et al. [8] and Sokooti et al. [14] aim at predicting IR uncertainty using machine learning techniques. Risholm et al. [11] presented a Bayesian approach to image registration, estimating the posterior distribution of the deformation field using a Markov Chain Monte-Carlo method. Hub et al. [6] proposed a local uncertainty estimation method by examining the variance of the similarity measure to local perturbations of the deformation field. Simpson et al. [12] presented a probabilistic IR framework that infers the appropriate level of regularization from the data, thereby also providing uncertainty estimates for the deformation field. However, none of these works focuses specifically on the uncertainty in IR due to the uncertainty in tuning parameters.

In this study, we propose a method to quantify the local IR uncertainty using an efficient surrogate modeling approach based on polynomial chaos expansion (PCE) [2]. Given a specified distribution on each input tuning parameter, this approach requires only a few image registration runs to characterize the distribution of output deformation estimates at each voxel. PCE is used for quantification of uncertainty of a process with regard to its inputs in many branches of engineering and science [17]. In our previous work [4], we explored the use of PCE to generate approximate IR results for different tuning parameters in real time, to facilitate interactive parameter tuning, but they did not evaluate the use of PCE for quantifying IR uncertainty. To the best of our knowledge, this is the first study where PCE is used to assess local IR uncertainty.

PCE models a process with one or more stochastic inputs using orthogonal polynomials with a compact representation. Modeling of the process is established by sampling the process outputs (here: deformation field) for a modest number of values of the input parameters (here: tuning parameters). Once the model is constructed, uncertainty of the output due to uncertainty in the input parameters is derived straightforwardly from the coefficients of the polynomials. Thanks to sparse grid sampling techniques [1,5,9], the PCE approach scales well with increasing dimension of the input parameter space.

2   Method

2.1   Uncertainty in Image Registration

The goal of IR is to estimate a spatial transformation $T(x)$ between the D-dimensional fixed image $F(x)$ and moving image $M(x)$. The transformation maps coordinates x from the fixed image domain to the moving image domain, such that the warped moving image $M(T(x))$ is aligned with the fixed image $F(x)$. IR is commonly formulated as a minimization problem:

$$\hat{T} = \arg\min_T C(T; F, M), \tag{1}$$

where $C(T; F, M)$ is a cost function that measures the dissimilarity between $F(x)$ and $M(T(x))$, and frequently also includes penalty/regularisation terms that promote desirable properties of the coordinate transformation T, such as smoothness or invertibility.

Almost any IR algorithm involves a number of user-defined tuning parameters, such as weights controlling the trade-off between dissimilarity and regularisation terms, settings of any smoothing filters used to preprocess the images, number of histogram bins to compute mutual information, and so on. These user-defined tuning parameters affect the solution $\hat{T}$. Denoting the tuning parameters by a vector p, we make this dependence explicit as follows:

$$\hat{T}_p = \arg\min_T C(T; F, M, p), \tag{2}$$

To establish reasonable values for p, it is common practice to perform some initial experiments on training data with a gold standard (e.g., corresponding landmarks or manual segmentations). However, the optimal value of p may differ from image to image, the gold standard usually has limited accuracy itself, and the size of the training data is often limited. Therefore, uncertainty in the optimal value of p remains, and this leads to uncertainty in $\hat{T}_p$. Our aim is to quantify the local uncertainty $\hat{T}_p(x)$ at each coordinate x.

2.2   Polynomial Chaos Expansion

Fundamentals of PCE were first introduced by Wiener [19] by pointing out that any second order random variable (Y) can be approximated by a superposition of polynomials of Gaussian random variables:

$$Y(X) \approx Y_{PCE}(X) = \sum_{k=0}^{K} c_k \psi_k(X), \tag{3}$$

where (Y_{PCE}) is the PCE approximation of Y, ψ_k are multivariate Hermite polynomials, c_k are their weighting coefficients, K is the number of polynomial basis functions which follows from the maximum allowed polynomial order, and X is an N-dimensional Gaussian random vector. The ψ_k's are members of the Hermite polynomial set and orthogonal to each other with respect to the Gaussian measure. The PCE method can be extended to support other random variable distributions for X as well, which lead to different choices of the polynomial sets [20]. Finding the coefficients c_k such that Y_{PCE} approximates the true value Y is the main objective of the method and they are determined using spectral projections as follows:

$$c_k = \frac{\langle Y(X), \psi_k(X) \rangle}{\langle \psi_k(X), \psi_k(X) \rangle} = \frac{\int ... \int Y(X)\psi_k(X)p(X)dX_1...dX_N}{\langle \psi_k(X), \psi_k(X) \rangle}. \tag{4}$$

Finding c_k can be computationally demanding especially for multiple input parameters (high dimension N of X), and therefore, may pose a problem for the feasibility of the method. However, the severity of the problem is considerably alleviated by harnessing sparse grid based numerical integration [1,5,9]. In these approaches, the sparsity of the grid is controlled by the "sparse grid level" setting [9]. Polynomial order and sparse grid level selection influence the accuracy of the PCE approximation and determine the number and location of sample points X required for the numerical integration in (4). The locations of sample points are fully determined by these parameters and by the distribution of X.

PCE construction is agnostic of the process $Y(X)$, and treats it as a black box function. Once the model Y_{PCE} has been trained by calculating the coefficients c_k, statistical moments of the output can be efficiently computed [17]. For example, taking the standard deviation as an uncertainty measure:

$$Std[Y] = \sqrt{E_X[Y_{PCE}^2] - E_X[Y_{PCE}]^2}. \tag{5}$$

Since $E_X[Y_{PCE}] = c_0$ and all ψ_k's are orthogonal to each other, Eq. 5 boils down to:

$$Std[Y] = \sqrt{\sum_{k=1}^{K} c_k^2 \langle \psi_k(X), \psi_k(X) \rangle}, \tag{6}$$

where $\langle \psi_k(X), \psi_k(X) \rangle$ is a projection of the polynomials with the same index, which is a constant that does not pose any computational overhead. Therefore, the uncertainty in Y due to uncertainty in X can be straightforwardly computed after the construction of the PCE model.

2.3   Local Image Registration Uncertainty Estimation with PCE

In our work, we are interested in quantifying the uncertainty in local transformation estimates $\hat{T}_p(x)$ due to uncertainty in the tuning parameters p, and we propose to use PCE for this purpose. For each voxel location x_v in the fixed image domain and for each dimension $i = 1 \dots D$, we construct an independent PCE model:

$$\hat{T}_p^i(\boldsymbol{x}_v) \approx \sum_{k=0}^{K} c_k^i(\boldsymbol{x}_v)\psi_k(\boldsymbol{p}). \qquad (7)$$

Here, it is assumed that the user has specified the distribution of $\boldsymbol{p}$, reflecting his/her prior knowledge on the feasible values of the tuning parameters, and has selected suitable values for the polynomial order and the sparse grid level. The coefficients $c_k^i(\boldsymbol{x}_v)$ are computed for all voxels as per Eq. 4, which requires the execution of a modest number of IRs for the samples of $\boldsymbol{p}$ indicated by the PCE algorithm.

Subsequently, for each voxel location $\boldsymbol{x}_v$ and dimension index i, the standard deviation is calculated as per Eq. 6

$$\sigma^i(\boldsymbol{x}_v) = Std[\hat{T}_p^i(\boldsymbol{x}_v)] = \sqrt{\sum_{k=1}^{K} c_k^i(\boldsymbol{x}_v)^2 \langle \psi_k(\boldsymbol{p}), \psi_k(\boldsymbol{p}) \rangle}. \qquad (8)$$

3 Experiments and Results

3.1 Dataset

7 pairs of abdominal CT images taken from 7 patients for ablation interventions are used for verification of the method. They were anonymized and acquired at Erasmus MC in 2014. Resolutions of images vary from $0.71\,\text{mm} \times 0.71\,\text{mm}$ to $0.84\,\text{mm} \times 0.84\,\text{mm}$ (501×492 to 512×512 in-plane resolution), 3–5 mm slice spacing and 1–2 mm slice thickness (16 to 70 slices). For each patient, we have one intra-operative CT, treated as fixed image, and one pre-operative CT, treated as moving image. Due to differences in patient position and breathing motion, large deformations may occur, and image registration is desired to improve image-guidance during the intervention.

3.2 Experiments

In our experiments, we implemented a parametric intensity-based IR method using mutual information (MI) as a dissimilarity measure in combination with two penalty terms P_1 and P_2. The IR can be mathematically represented by the following optimization problem:

$$\hat{T}_p = \arg\min_{T} MI(\boldsymbol{T}; F, M) + 2^{p_1} P_1(\boldsymbol{T}) + 2^{p_2} P_2(\boldsymbol{T}), \qquad (9)$$

with $\boldsymbol{p} = (p_1, p_2)$ the vector of $N = 2$ tuning parameters that serve as weighting coefficients for the penalty terms P_1 and P_2. In the experiments, we chose *transform bending energy* [16] and *point-to-surface* [3] penalty terms for P_1 and P_2, respectively. Bending energy is an often used measure to promote smoothness

of the deformation. The point-to-surface penalty term drives manually annotated points in the fixed image onto the liver surface in the moving image,
and was proposed in [3] as an efficient way to incorporate user-provided constraints into the registration process. For the experiments in this work, we manually segmented the liver surface in the moving image, and annotated around
75 points on the liver surface in the fixed image, as suggested by [3]. For
the transformation we used a B-spline free-form deformation model with an
isotropic control point spacing of 10 mm. Equation (9) was solved with a quasi-
Newton Broyden−Fletcher−Goldfarb−Shanno optimization method. No registration masks or deformation field boundary conditions were applied.

To assign a suitable distribution to the penalty weights p_1 and p_2, we performed a one-dimensional grid search for each of these parameters, optimizing
the Dice overlaps between manual liver segmentations. Mean and standard deviation of the optimal values for p_1 and p_2 obtained for the 7 image pairs were
computed and used as the center and spread parameters of the Gaussian distributions of p_1 ($\mu = 6$, $\sigma^2 = 4$) and p_2 ($\mu = -9$, $\sigma^2 = 1$).

In the experiments, we select respectively 4 and 3 for polynomial order and
sparse grid level for the construction of the PCE model. Given this setting, 17
sample points (i.e., IR runs) are required to establish the model. Using the outcome of these IRs, corresponding deformation fields are generated, PCE models
are constructed, and finally the uncertainty map $\sigma(x)$ is obtained. In order to
assess the accuracy of the uncertainty map, we compare it with the result of
a brute-force Monte Carlo simulation using 225 IR runs. Both qualitative and
quantitative results are presented.

To implement the PCE model, we used the open source OpenPC library
[10,18].

3.3 Results

Figure 1 shows example slices of Dataset1. Panels (a) and (c) present the fixed
and moving images, respectively. The moving image after registration is shown
on panel (b). The deformed image was obtained using the 'optimal' setting of p
(i.e., at the mean of the distribution). PCE and Monte-Carlo simulation based
uncertainty maps of this registration are presented in Fig. 2 for x, y and z directions. It appears that results of the PCE are highly similar to Monte-Carlo
simulation based uncertainty estimates. PCE effectively captures small details
in the reference estimates and the performance is consistent in all directions.
Comparing the local uncertainty estimates with the image information at the
corresponding locations in the fixed and deformed moving image (Figs. 1(a) and
(b)), we observe that the uncertainty is higher in the background and lower
near salient structures such as the spine. Off note, the uncertainty in y-direction
(Fig. 2(d)) shows a clear minimum at the anterior skin/air interface.

In Table 1, mean standard deviations of the Monte-Carlo simulation (σ_{mc})
and PCE model (σ_{pce}) and root mean square of their differences (Δ_σ) over all
voxels and directions are presented for 7 datasets. The results are in mm scale. In
interpreting these results, it should be noted that we did not apply any boundary

conditions or image region mask for the implemented registrations. Therefore, there occur large uncertainties around the boundaries of the image volume and the regions outside the patient body where the image lacks salient structures, as could be seen in Fig. 2. These large values explain the relatively high mean uncertainties. Nonetheless, the root mean square different Δ_σ is consistently low compared to the mean uncertainty, indicating that the efficient PCE matches the brute-force Monte-Carlo estimate.

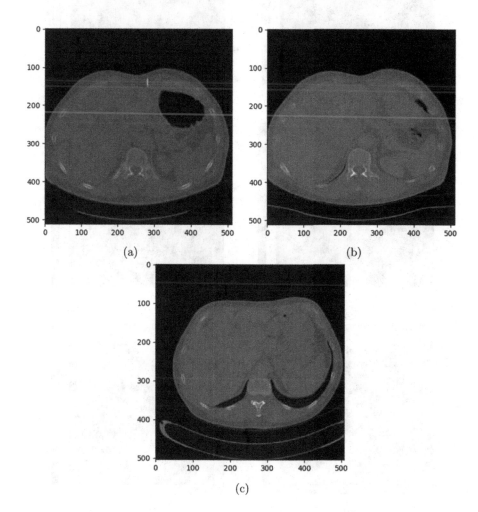

Fig. 1. Fixed image (a), registered moving image (b) and moving image (c).

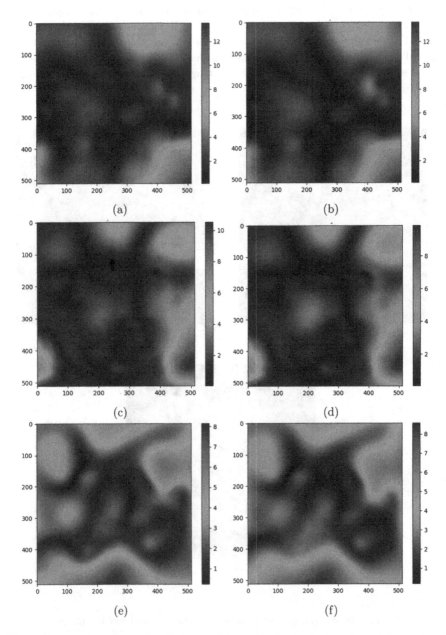

Fig. 2. Uncertainty maps obtained using Monte-Carlo simulations for x (a), y (c) and z (e) directions and PCE model for x (b), y (d) and z (f) directions. The colour bar shows local IR uncertainty $\sigma^i(\boldsymbol{x})$ in mm units. (Color figure online)

Table 1. Mean value of the uncertainties $\sigma(x)$ over all voxels in each image, as computed with the Monte-Carlo simulation (σ_{mc}), and with the proposed PCE approach (σ_{PCE}). The last column shows the root mean square voxel-wise difference between the two estimates (Δ_σ).

Dataset	σ_{mc} in mm	σ_{pce} in mm	Δ_σ in mm
1	5.44	5.50	0.58
2	5.26	4.85	0.57
3	4.36	5.04	0.93
4	4.32	4.90	0.91
5	4.31	4.53	0.57
6	9.06	9.37	1.66
7	5.16	5.16	1.20

4 Discussion and Conclusion

Most image registration methods involve user-defined parameters which need to be tuned for the sake registration performance. However, in general there is no universal value for these parameters working well for all cases, and optimal values of these parameters may change even for different image pairs with the same registration setup. Therefore, optimal values of these parameters bear uncertainties which in turn cause uncertainties in the registration results. In this study, we introduced a method for quantification of the local IR uncertainties, based on a computationally efficient polynomial chaos expansion (PCE) approach.

In experiments on 7 abdominal CT image pairs, we evaluated the accuracy of the uncertainty estimates by PCE, by comparing them to the results of an (expensive) Monte-Carlo simulation. The Monte-Carlo simulation was realized with 225 samples (i.e., IR executions at different settings of the tuning parameters), whereas the proposed PCE method only required 17 IR runs, making it much more efficient. The results show that the local IR uncertainty estimates by both methods are highly comparable, indicating the validity of the proposed PCE approach.

In future work, we will extend the evaluation by including more tuning parameters, such as B-spline control point spacing, step size of the optimization method, number of histogram bins used in the computation of mutual information, multi-scale image pyramid settings, and so on. Moreover, we will investigate the use of 'Sobol indices', as a way to decompose the variance of the IR estimates into fractions that can be attributed to individual tuning parameters or to interactions of tuning parameters [13].

References

1. Blatman, G., Sudret, B.: Adaptive sparse polynomial chaos expansion based on least angle regression. J. Comput. Phys. **230**(6), 2345–2367 (2011)
2. Crestaux, T., Matre, O.L., Martinez, J.M.: Polynomial chaos expansion for sensitivity analysis. Reliab. Eng. Syst. Saf. **94**(7), 1161–1172 (2009)
3. Gunay, G., Luu, M.H., Moelker, A., van Walsum, T., Klein, S.: Semiautomated registration of pre- and intraoperative CT for image-guided percutaneous liver tumor ablation interventions. Med. Phys. **44**(7), 3718–3725 (2017)
4. Gunay, G., van der Voort, S., Luu, M.H., Moelker, A., Klein, S.: Parameter sensitivity analysis in medical image registration algorithms using polynomial chaos expansions. In: Descoteaux, M., Maier-Hein, L., Franz, A., Jannin, P., Collins, D.L., Duchesne, S. (eds.) MICCAI 2017. LNCS, vol. 10433, pp. 335–343. Springer, Cham (2017). https://doi.org/10.1007/978-3-319-66182-7_39
5. Hu, C., Youn, B.D.: Adaptive-sparse polynomial chaos expansion for reliability analysis and design of complex engineering systems. Struct. Multidiscip. Optim. **43**(3), 419–442 (2011)
6. Hub, M., Kessler, M.L., Karger, C.P.: A stochastic approach to estimate the uncertainty involved in B-spline image registration. IEEE Trans. Med. Imaging **28**(11), 1708–1716 (2009)
7. Kybic, J.: Bootstrap resampling for image registration uncertainty estimation without ground truth. IEEE Trans. Image Process. **19**(1), 64–73 (2010)
8. Muenzing, S.E., van Ginneken, B., Murphy, K., Pluim, J.P.: Supervised quality assessment of medical image registration: application to intra-patient CT lung registration. Med. Image Anal. **16**, 1521–1531 (2012)
9. Perko, Z., Gilli, L., Lathouwers, D., Kloosterman, J.L.: Grid and basis adaptive polynomial chaos techniques for sensitivity and uncertainty analysis. J. Comput. Phys. **260**, 54–84 (2014)
10. Perko, Z., van der Voort, S.R., van de Water, S., Hartman, C.M.H., Hoogeman, M., Lathouwers, D.: Fast and accurate sensitivity analysis of IMPT treatment plans using polynomial chaos expansion. Phys. Med. Biol. **61**(12), 4646 (2016)
11. Risholm, P., Pieper, S., Samset, E., Wells, W.M.: Summarizing and visualizing uncertainty in non-rigid registration. In: Jiang, T., Navab, N., Pluim, J.P.W., Viergever, M.A. (eds.) MICCAI 2010. LNCS, vol. 6362, pp. 554–561. Springer, Heidelberg (2010). https://doi.org/10.1007/978-3-642-15745-5_68
12. Simpson, I.J., Schnabel, J.A., Groves, A.R., Andersson, J.L., Woolrich, M.W.: Probabilistic inference of regularisation in non-rigid registration. NeuroImage **59**(3), 2438–2451 (2012)
13. Sobol, I.M.: Global sensitivity indices for nonlinear mathematical models and their Monte Carlo estimates. Math. Comput. Simul. **55**(1), 271–280 (2001)
14. Sokooti, H., Saygili, G., Glocker, B., Lelieveldt, B.P.F., Staring, M.: Accuracy estimation for medical image registration using regression forests. In: Ourselin, S., Joskowicz, L., Sabuncu, M.R., Unal, G., Wells, W. (eds.) MICCAI 2016. LNCS, vol. 9902, pp. 107–115. Springer, Cham (2016). https://doi.org/10.1007/978-3-319-46726-9_13
15. Sotiras, A., Davatzikos, C., Paragios, N.: Deformable medical image registration: a survey. IEEE Trans. Med. Imaging **32**(7), 1153–1190 (2013)
16. Staring, M., Klein, S., Pluim, J.P.W.: A rigidity penalty term for nonrigid registration. Med. Phys. **34**(11), 4098–4108 (2007)

17. Sudret, B.: Global sensitivity analysis using polynomial chaos expansions. Reliab. Eng. Syst. Saf. **93**(7), 964–979 (2008)
18. van der Voort, S., van de Water, S., Perk, Z., Heijmen, B., Lathouwers, D., Hoogeman, M.: Robustness recipes for minimax robust optimization in intensity modulated proton therapy for oropharyngeal cancer patients. Int. J. Radiat. Oncol. Biol. Phys. **95**(1), 163–170 (2016)
19. Wiener, N.: The homogeneous chaos. Am. J. Math. **60**(4), 897–936 (1938)
20. Xiu, D., Karniadakis, G.E.: The Wiener-Askey polynomial chaos for stochastic differential equations. SIAM J. Sci. Comput. **24**(2), 619–644 (2002)

Author Index

Printed in the United States
By Bookmasters